# *SELF*
# HEALTH

"Reverse Chronic Disease, Restore Your Vitality and
Transform Your Life: One Choice at a Time"

By Dr. Fabrizio Mancini

This book is intended solely for educational and informational purposes. It is not intended to diagnose, treat, cure, or prevent any disease, and it is not a substitute for professional medical advice,

Some topics covered in this book involve emerging areas of science. Readers are advised that such content may reflect early-stage findings and ongoing debate and should not be considered definitive or universally endorsed by the broader medical community.

Names, characters, and events portrayed in this publication may be fictitious or used with permission for illustrative purposes. Any resemblance to real persons, living or dead, is purely coincidental unless explicitly stated.

The authors and publishers are not responsible for any adverse effects or consequences resulting from the use of any suggestions, recommendations, or procedures described in this book. By reading this book, you agree to assume full responsibility for your decisions regarding your health and wellness.

If you are experiencing a medical emergency or have serious health concerns, contact your physician or emergency services immediately.

**Book Layout and Design** by Shefa Rumby
**Printed in the United States of America**

**ISBN**: [979-8-9927264-4-2] Hardback
**ISBN**: [979-8-9927264-3-5] Paperback
**ISBN**: [979-8-9927264-2-8] eBook

# Table of Contents

# Discover Your Chronic Disease Risk Score

Are you at risk for chronic disease? Understanding your risk is the first critical step toward reclaiming your health and preventing chronic illness.

**Take the FREE Chronic Disease Risk Assessment**

By scanning the QR code below, you'll receive:

- **Personalized Risk Score:** Instantly find out your current risk level for chronic disease.
- **Customized Recommendations:** Get tailored, practical steps you can take today to significantly reduce your risk and improve your health.
- **Expert Insights:** Access proven strategies from leading health professionals to help you end chronic disease for good.
- **Exclusive Resources:** Benefit from Dr. Fab's *How to Read a Food Label, 30 Delicious Recipes for Chronic Disease, 10 Secrets for Ending Chronic Disease* and much more.

Scan the QR code NOW to take control of your health and start your journey to wellness.

www.drfabmancini.com/exclusive-resources

Act now: your future self will be grateful! Don't forget to scan the QR code for each member of your family, and feel free to share it with your loved ones!

# PREFACE:

## The Power to Change Your Health and Life

What if I told you that many of today's most common chronic diseases, heart disease, diabetes, obesity, cognitive decline, and autoimmune disorders, aren't just random misfortunes, but conditions that may be prevented, reversed, and even *eliminated* altogether?

What if I told you that true healing doesn't come from a pill, a medical procedure, or the latest healthcare breakthrough, but from something far more powerful and within your control: *your* daily choices?

For too long, we've been taught that chronic disease is inevitable. We've been told that aging means suffering, that our genes determine our fate, and that medication is the only way to manage illness. But science tells a different story: one of *hope, empowerment,* and *transformation.*

Chronic disease is not a life sentence; it's a wake-up call. Imagine carrying a heavy backpack filled with rocks, each one representing a burden on your health: chronic stress, poor diet, toxins, lack of sleep, emotional trauma, or unresolved infections. At first, the weight seems manageable, but over time, it grows heavier. Your body starts to strain: your posture suffers, your energy drains, and every step becomes harder.

This is how chronic disease develops: not as a sudden, overwhelming burden, but as the slow accumulation of stressors that wear you down. Conventional treatments often act as a walking stick, helping you cope while still carrying the weight. But *true healing* comes from stopping, opening the backpack, and removing the rocks one by one:

- **The processed food rock**? Replace it with nutrient-dense foods rich in vitamins, minerals, and antioxidants that will nourish your body. Include fresh vegetables, fruits, high-quality proteins, healthy fats, and fiber-rich foods to fuel your body and promote healing. Ditch artificial additives, excess sugar, and unhealthy oils which contribute to inflammation and disease.

- **The toxin rock**? Remove it by supporting detox pathways and reducing environmental exposures. Drink plenty of clean water, eat foods that enhance your bodily functions (such as garlic and turmeric), and reduce exposure to harmful chemicals in household products, skincare, and plastics. Be mindful of your body's surroundings.

- **The stress rock?** Lighten this through mindfulness, movement, and emotional healing. Practice different ways to reduce your mental strain and better process your emotions and reactions, such as meditation, deep breathing, or journaling. Release built-up tension through physical activities such as yoga, walking, or strength training.

- **The sleep deprivation rock?** Swap it for restorative rest that allows your body to repair itself. Establish a consistent sleep schedule, and optimize your sleep environment with a dark, cool, and quiet room. Proper sleep quality gives your body the best chance to function at its best.

With each rock you remove, the burden lifts. Your steps feel lighter, your energy returns, and you rediscover the freedom of moving without unnecessary weight holding you back.

*Self-health* isn't about adding more to the load; it's about letting go of what no longer serves you. By addressing the root causes, you can move forward freely, unburdened by the weight of chronic disease threatening to slow you down.

In my 35 years of clinical experience, I've seen that it's the small, sustainable changes we make every day that lead to the most profound transformations in health and life.

## The Moment Everything Changed

I have dedicated over three decades working in the wellness field, treating thousands of patients, lecturing around the world, and sharing the truth about healing. I chose to become a Doctor of Chiropractic rather than a medical doctor because I wanted to empower people with the understanding that the body is a self-healing, self-regulating organism.

Our bodies are made up of intricate systems and organs designed to work in harmony to maintain health. From the beginning, my mission was to focus on preventing disease by addressing its root causes, not simply managing symptoms. After more than 30 years of caring for patients, my passion for this approach has only grown stronger. Today, emerging science continues to validate what I've witnessed first-hand throughout my career: that true healing begins from within.

But the moment that truly changed everything for me didn't happen in a clinic or on a global stage; it happened in a simple conversation with a patient. She was a woman in her 40s, exhausted, overweight, and reliant on multiple medications. She looked at me with tired eyes and said, "Maybe this is just how life is now." Her words broke my heart, not because she was sick, but because she had given up hope. And I know she's not alone. Maybe you've felt that way too, like your body is failing you and no one is listening. If so, I want you to know I see you. I believe you. And I believe in your ability to heal.

That woman made one small change, she swapped soda for water. Encouraged by that step, she began adding more whole foods to her diet and walking daily. Those small changes became her norm, and within months, her life was completely transformed. Her energy soared, she lost weight effortlessly, and most importantly, she reversed her diabetes diagnosis. She did *not* do this with a prescription, but instead with *consistent, healthy* daily actions.

That experience lit a fire in me that has never gone out. I'm not just passionate about health, I'm relentless in helping people find real answers to their health frustrations. If you've ever felt stuck, overwhelmed, or unheard, know that there is hope. Healing is possible. And it often starts with just one small step.

This book was inspired by stories like hers: real people who took control of their health and transformed their lives through simple, intentional changes.

People who stopped relying on quick fixes or medications alone, and instead focused on nourishing their bodies with *healthy foods*, prioritizing deep, restorative *sleep*, shifting their *mindset* towards healing, and *moving daily* in ways that felt good for their body.

This self-health book is for those individuals who refused to accept chronic illness as their fate and instead chose a path for lasting well-being.

## Why This Book? Why Now?

We are in the midst of a health crisis, not because we lack access to information, but because we've prioritized everything *but* our well-being. The **SELF HEALTH** movement begins with a powerful truth: the best way to self-help is to **self-health**.

True success in life, work, and relationships starts with the foundation of a healthy body and mind. According to a 2023 study published in *The Lancet Public Health*, individuals who adopted healthy lifestyle behaviors, such as quality sleep, balanced nutrition, stress management, and regular movement, reduced their risk of developing chronic diseases by up to **74%**, and increased life expectancy by nearly **10 years**, even in the presence of genetic risk factors.

This evidence reinforces what this book stands for: **self-health isn't just about avoiding disease, it's about being intentional with your daily choices** to create a thriving, resilient life.

Every chapter in this book is designed to help you take back control, not just of your health, but of your entire future, because when health becomes your top priority, everything else improves.

The reality is, this health crisis has reached unprecedented proportions. In the United States alone:

- **6 in 10 adults** suffer from a chronic disease (CDC, 2023).
- **1 in 3 children** is overweight or obese, setting the stage for future health struggles.
- **Rates of Alzheimer's, heart disease, diabetes, and autoimmune diseases** are rising at an alarming pace, affecting millions and placing an increasing burden on individuals, families, and the healthcare system.

And yet, **90%** of these diseases are driven by lifestyle choices.

This means that 90% of chronic disease is within our control. The food we eat, the way we move, how we manage stress, the quality of our sleep, and the environment we create all play a powerful role in our health.

This book is not just about disease prevention, it's about *creating lasting health.* It's about learning how to use food as medicine, how to move your body in ways that promote healing, how to master stress and sleep to restore balance, how to detox from harmful toxins, and how to reprogram your mindset for vitality. It's about understanding that true wellness isn't just the absence of illness; it's the presence of energy, resilience, and a thriving body and mind.

## The Choice is Yours

Every day, you make choices that either feed disease or fight it. This book is designed to be your *roadmap to transformation.* Guiding you step by step toward a healthier, fuller life. With this book you will:

- **Learn the truth** about why chronic disease has skyrocketed, and your best chance to reverse it.

- **Uncover the hidden factors** that are sabotaging your health, and some simple, accessible ways to beat them.

- **Discover practical, actionable steps** you can start implementing right away, because even small, consistent changes can create powerful, lasting results.

Are You Ready?

If you're ready to take back control, restore your energy, and break free from chronic disease, this book is for you. Your health is your most valuable asset, and the best part? *You have the power to change it.* The journey to *self-health* begins now, and the choice is yours.

Let's get started.

# INTRODUCTION:

## Ending the Epidemic We Created: The Silent Crisis of Chronic Disease

Imagine waking up every morning feeling exhausted, sluggish, and weighed down by pain. Now, understand that this has become the reality for millions of people worldwide. Chronic disease, once a rarity, has become an epidemic, affecting **6 in 10 adults** in the U.S. alone. Heart disease, diabetes, obesity, autoimmune disorders, and cognitive decline are no longer diseases limited to the elderly; they are increasingly affecting younger generations at an alarming rate.

Here's the truth most people don't realize: chronic disease is *largely preventable* and, in many cases, *reversible*. We've been conditioned to believe that disease is simply a matter of bad luck or genetics. But the reality is that 90% of chronic disease is driven by lifestyle choices: what we eat, how we move, how we sleep, and how we manage stress. Science backs this up time and time again, yet many people still turn to medication as their only solution.

**Let's be clear**: The current medical model is not designed to cure chronic disease. It's designed to manage symptoms, often keeping people dependent on medications for life. That is not healthcare, that's sick care. An integrative approach to health can help support better outcomes.

## The Power of Self-Health in Shaping Our Health

Imagine your body as a house that has been neglected for years: leaky pipes, a cracked foundation, and faulty wiring. Chronic disease is like the result of this neglect. Reversing it isn't about just slapping on a coat of paint (medications to mask symptoms); it's about going deeper, fixing the foundation (gut health), rewiring the electricity (nervous system), and upgrading the plumbing (detoxification).

True healing happens when we restore the house from the inside out, not patch it with temporary fixes. When we focus on rebuilding the foundation and systems that support the body, we create a strong, resilient structure that can thrive.

In the past 35 years, my mission has always been the same: to help people reclaim their health and end unnecessary suffering and expense. Through my work, I've witnessed countless individuals have great improvements in symptoms associated with chronic disease, not through costly medications or surgeries, but through simple, everyday choices.

The power to heal lies within our daily decisions, for example, in my years of experience I have worked with:

- A woman in her 40s who put into remission her type 2 diabetes diagnosis by changing her diet and lifestyle.

- A father of three who went from relying on daily pain medication to being completely pain-free by incorporating regular movement, chiropractic care and adopting an anti-inflammatory diet.

- A woman who significantly improved her symptoms from early signs of Alzheimer's by changing her diet, adding supplements and prioritizing sleep.

Every day, we make thousands of small decisions that either move us closer to disease or toward better health. The food we eat, the thoughts we think, the time we spend outdoors, each of these choices shapes our biology. And so, the power to influence our health lies in the decisions we make each moment. To reestablish control of our health we must shift from a reactionary approach, waiting until disease develops, to a proactive approach, where we prevent and reverse disease before it controls our lives.

# The Compound Effect of Daily Choices

Think of your health like a savings account. Every positive decision (eating a whole food meal, exercising, getting restful sleep) is like making a deposit. Every negative decision (eating processed foods, staying inactive, dealing with chronic stress) is like making a withdrawal. Over time, your balance either grows or depletes based on the choices you make. These decisions might seem abstract at first, but the proof (or profit) is in plain sight:

- **Food as health profits:** Eating real, whole foods lower inflammation, stabilizes blood sugar, and supports healing. A Mediterranean-style diet has been linked to a 30% lower risk of heart disease (NEJM, 2022).

- **Movement as health profits:** Just 30 minutes of walking daily reduces the risk of chronic disease by 50% (JAMA, 2021).

- **Sleep as health profits:** Sleep deprivation increases the risk of obesity, diabetes, and Alzheimer's, yet most people don't prioritize sleep (National Sleep Foundation, 2023).

- **Stress Reduction as health profits:** Chronic stress raises cortisol levels, fueling inflammation and weight gain. Simple breathing exercises can lower blood pressure and improve immunity (APA, 2023).

# Why the Old Medical Model is Failing Us

The current healthcare system isn't focused on preventing or reversing disease; it's focused on managing symptoms with drugs.

Let's take a closer look at some shocking facts:

- The average American takes **four** prescription medications daily (CDC, 2022).

- **90%** of healthcare costs go toward treating chronic disease (CDC, 2024).

- Despite spending more on healthcare than any other country, the U.S. ranks among the sickest developed nations (The Lancet, 2022).

- The U.S. health care system spent a staggering $603 billion on prescription drugs, before accounting for rebates, with $421 billion of that amount spent on retail drugs (HHS, 2021).

The truth is, the system isn't designed to keep us healthy; it's designed to keep us dependent. Most doctors aren't trained in nutrition, lifestyle medicine, or holistic healing; they are trained to diagnose and prescribe. Pharmaceutical companies profit when we stay sick, the food industry thrives when we consume highly processed, addictive foods, and insurance companies benefit from keeping people trapped in a cycle of dependence.

But here's the good news: *You don't have to play their game.* You have the power to take control of your health and make choices that break the cycle, permanently stepping out of a system that profits from your sickness.

## The Choices We Make Today Will Shape Our Children's Future

If we don't change course now, and do so quickly, the next generation will face even greater challenges than we do. They are already facing unprecedented challenges related to chronic disease, including **1 in 5 children** already struggling with obesity (CDC, 2023), and an increase in **type 2 diabetes** diagnoses, a disease once considered only present in adults. The bleak truth is that children today are already expected to live shorter lives than their parents.

As a parent or caregiver, you have the power to rewrite this story. You are the gatekeeper of your home's health. You decide what foods are purchased, how much movement is encouraged, and how stress is managed. If you take the lead, your family will follow, and that ripple effect can transform generations to come. The choices you make today can ensure a healthier, brighter future for your loved ones.

## Your Next Steps: How to Take Immediate Action

Transformation doesn't happen overnight, but it does start with small, intentional steps. Here are some easy, accessible steps that can start doing today in order to start changing tomorrow:

- **Swap one processed meal for a whole food meal**: Try fresh, nutrient-dense options instead of processed starches and unnecessary sugars.

- **Move your body for 30 minutes:** Whether it's a walk, some stretching, or dancing to your favorite song while doing things around the house.

- **Turn off all screens 30 minutes before bed**: This is imperative to improving your sleep and allowing your body to rest and recharge for the next day.

- **Drink more water**: Try to cut back on sugary drinks and replace them with water to hydrate and nourish your body.

- **Take five deep breaths right now**: This is a mindful practice that reduces stress and calms your mind.

Small changes add up over time, and you have more power than you think. This is just the beginning of your journey to a healthier, disease-free life. Are you ready to reclaim your health? *The choice is yours.*

# PART I:
# Chronic Disease – Uncovering the Root Causes

# Chapter 1:
# Understanding Chronic Disease:
# Are You at Risk?

## Chronic Disease – The Root Causes of Modern Illness

**Chronic diseases kill more people than all infectious diseases, accidents, and natural disasters combined; yet 90% are preventable.**

Imagine waking up one day feeling trapped in your own body: exhausted, in pain, and reliant on medications. That was Lisa's reality. At 42, she was diagnosed with type 2 diabetes, hypertension, and joint pain so severe she struggled to play with her kids. Doctors prescribed medication after medication, but none addressed the root cause. Frustrated, Lisa took control of her health. She changed her diet, moved her body daily, began using acupuncture and managed her stress. Within a year, she was off all medications, full of energy, and reclaiming the life she thought she lost.

Building on our earlier "body as a house" analogy, imagine a tiny leak in your home's plumbing. At first, it seems minor, just a few drops of water here and there. But over time, that leak weakens the foundation, leading to mold, rot, and structural damage. By the time the issue becomes obvious, the damage is extensive and costly to repair.

Chronic disease works the same way. Small daily choices (poor diet, lack of movement, chronic stress, and toxin exposure) may not seem harmful at first. But over the years, they silently erode your health, leading to major breakdowns like diabetes, heart disease, and systemic inflammation. This is because chronic disease doesn't just *happen*, it's built through our daily choices.

The good news? Just as fixing a leak early can prevent disaster, making small, intentional health changes today can stop the damage and restore your body before it reaches the breaking point. Your health isn't just about avoiding disease; it's about building a strong, resilient foundation for a thriving life, and this book will act as the roadmap to building that foundation and reversing any existing damage.

## What is Chronic Disease?

Chronic diseases, such as diabetes, heart disease, autoimmune disorders, and obesity, are now the leading causes of death and disability worldwide. Unlike acute illnesses like infections or injuries, these conditions develop gradually, persist for years, and often require ongoing management. However, many chronic diseases are not only *preventable* but also *reversible* with the right lifestyle changes.

Information about chronic diseases comes from countless sources: medical professionals, online articles, social media, and word of mouth. Unfortunately, this flood of information often leads to widespread myths, misconceptions, and misinformation. Here are a few common examples:

## Common Myths vs. Reality

| Myth | Reality |
|---|---|
| Chronic disease is just a result of aging. | Many chronic diseases are lifestyle-driven, not age-dependent. Conditions like type 2 diabetes, heart disease, and even cognitive decline, once considered diseases of old age, are now appearing in people as young as their 30s and 40s. |
| If my parents had it, I will too. | Genetics load the gun, but lifestyle pulls the trigger. Your DNA is not your destiny. By making intentional, healthy choices, you have the power to prevent, manage, |

| | and even reverse many chronic diseases, regardless of your genetic background. |
|---|---|
| Medication is the only way to manage chronic disease. | Medications manage symptoms, but they rarely address root causes. They act like a bandage, masking the problem rather than solving it. True healing comes from lifestyle interventions. |

## The Hidden Impact: Chronic Disease as the Leading Cause of Death and Disability

Just as misinformation surrounds chronic diseases, their true impact on the population is often misunderstood or downplayed. The reality is alarming:

- According to the World Health Organization (WHO), chronic diseases account for **71%** of all global deaths.

- In the U.S., **6 in 10 adults** have at least one chronic disease, and **4 in 10** have two or more.

- Chronic diseases drive **90%** of healthcare costs, despite being largely preventable.

Beyond statistics, chronic disease **steals quality of life**: causing fatigue, pain, dependency on medications, and lost productivity. The burden extends beyond individuals, affecting families, workplaces, and healthcare systems worldwide.

## Acute Illness vs. Chronic Illness: A Side-by-Side Comparison

| Acute Illness | Chronic Disease |
| --- | --- |
| Sudden onset (flu, broken bone) | Develops gradually over time |
| Short-term, (weeks/months) | Long-lasting, often lifetime |
| Clear cause (infection, injury) | Multifactorial causes (diet, stress, toxins) |
| Often curable with treatment | Requires management with some Lifestyle changes |

Modern medicine excels at treating acute conditions: antibiotics cure infections, surgeries repair injuries, and emergency care saves lives. However, when it comes to *chronic* disease, the conventional medical approach often falls short.

Instead of addressing the *root causes*, it primarily focuses on *managing symptoms* through medications.

## How the System Profits from Chronic Disease

Chronic disease is a major driver of healthcare costs, and much of the system is structured around managing, not reversing, these conditions. Pharmaceutical companies generate significant revenue from long-term medication use, while the food industry benefits from the widespread consumption of ultra-processed foods linked to obesity, diabetes, and heart disease. Insurance models often reimburse ongoing treatment over prevention, reinforcing this cycle.

While these industries play important roles, their priorities may not always align with long-term healing. That's why it's essential for individuals to be informed, ask questions, and explore integrative approaches that support true health, by addressing root causes, not just symptoms. Prevention, lifestyle change, and holistic care can empower people to take charge of their well-being and pursue better outcomes.

## How Modern Lifestyles Are Fueling the Epidemic

Our ancestors thrived on natural movement, whole foods, and a deep connection to nature. Their lifestyles naturally supported health and vitality. Today's society, by comparison, has created a perfect storm for chronic disease:

**Ultra-Processed Diets & Sugar Overload:**

- The modern diet is filled with refined carbs, unhealthy fats, and artificial additives, leading to inflammation and insulin resistance.
- A study in *The Journal of the American Medical Association (JAMA)* found that added sugars **significantly increase** the risk of cardiovascular disease mortality.

**Sedentary Living:**

- Most people sit for **8+ hours daily**, leading to metabolic dysfunction, weakened muscles, and poor circulation.
- Research from *The Lancet* found that inactivity is as harmful to the body as smoking.

**Chronic Stress & Sleep Deprivation:**

- Chronic stress raises cortisol levels, fueling inflammation, weight gain, and immune dysfunction.
- Poor sleep **disrupts hormones**, increasing the risk of diabetes, obesity, and heart disease.

**Toxins & Gut Microbiome Imbalance:**

- Daily exposure to pesticides, plastics, air pollution, and heavy metals overwhelms the body's detox systems.
- Gut imbalances have been linked to obesity, diabetes, autoimmune disease, and even mental health disorders.

## Your 30-Day Action Plan: Reclaim Your Health Step-by-Step

Chronic disease doesn't develop overnight, and neither does healing. Healing takes time, but it starts with *small steps*. Whether it's swapping one processed meal for a whole food option, adding 10 minutes of movement to your day, or getting an extra hour of sleep, each positive choice builds momentum.

Let's start with the first month, week-by-week.

Here are some buildable and accessible steps to take on your first month's journey to total wellness:

**WEEK 1: Upgrade Your Diet**

- **Swap out processed foods for whole, nutrient-dense foods.** For example, swap processed deli meats for grilled chicken, turkey, or salmon. Swap chips and crackers for raw nuts and seeds.

- **Reduce sugar and refined carbs.** For example, swap rice and white bread for quinoa and whole grain. Swap sugary breakfast cereals for oatmeal.

- **Drink cleaner, filtered water.** Reduce sugary soda and juices and stay better hydrated and energized with more daily water intake.

## WEEK 2: Move More

- **Aim for 30 minutes of activity daily**: Walking, strength training, and yoga are all great examples.
- **Take frequent breaks from sitting**. If you work at a desk all day, stand up and stretch every hour.

## WEEK 3: Prioritize Sleep & Stress Management

- **Get 7-9 hours of quality sleep per night**. Stick to a regular schedule of going to bed and waking up the same hours every night and avoid screen time 30-60 minutes before bedtime.
- **Practice ways to naturally reduce stress.** For example, deep breathing, meditation, and nature walks. Even 5-10 minutes of daily meditation can go a long way in reducing overall stress levels.

## WEEK 4: Reduce Toxin Exposure & Build Community

- **Choose organic foods when possible.** When shopping, look for the USDA Organic label, choose a local farmers' market, or consider growing your own herbs and vegetables at home.

- **Use non-toxic household & personal care products**. Try natural alternatives to cleaning products, such as vinegar, baking soda, or castile soap. Choose fragrance- and paraben-free skincare products.

- **Surround yourself with positive, health-conscious individuals**. Find a like-minded community, whether that's joining a fitness group, seeking out a positive role model, or prioritizing healthy activities with friends.

You don't have to wait for permission to take back your life. Healing is in your hands, and every choice you make moves you closer to vitality or disease. The decision is yours. I've spent decades studying, researching, and applying these principles, not just in my practice, but also in my own life. This book is my way of giving you the tools to reclaim your health and step into the life you were meant to live.

### Next Up

In **Chapter 2**, we'll uncover the hidden factors driving chronic disease: many of which are overlooked in conventional medicine. You'll learn how these disruptors impact your health and, more importantly, how you can take back control starting today.

# Chapter 2:
# Why We Are Sick: How Lifestyle Fuels Chronic Illness

Did You Know? The Modern World is Making Us Sick

**Six in ten U.S. adults have at least one chronic disease, and four in ten have two or more; yet most of these conditions are preventable.**

At 50, Michael woke up every day feeling exhausted, sluggish, and dependent on medications. Diagnosed with high blood pressure, obesity, and early signs of fatty liver disease, he believed genetics had sealed his fate, until he decided to take back control. By changing his diet, exercising daily, and managing stress, Michael significantly improved every one of his symptoms from his conditions within a year. If he could do it, so can *you*.

Imagine a thriving forest where every tree, plant, and organism work in harmony to maintain balance. Now, picture a slow but steady poisoning of that ecosystem: polluted water, depleted soil, and toxic air disrupting its natural rhythms.

Over time, the trees weaken, the soil erodes, and disease spreads. This is exactly what happens to our bodies.

True healing isn't about masking the damage with more chemicals: it's about eliminating the source of the pollution, clearing out toxins, and restoring balance. *Your* body is that ecosystem, and you have the power to bring it back to health.

But you might wonder, how did we get here? Where did the poison come from, and how can we prevent it from seeping back in to contaminate the foundation of our health? To truly heal, we must first understand the hidden forces that have led to this imbalance. Only then can we take the necessary steps to restore, protect, and sustain our well-being for the long term.

## How We Got Here: The Root Causes of Chronic Disease

Chapter 1 introduced how our ancestors lived in sync with nature: eating whole, real foods, moving daily, sleeping in alignment with natural rhythms, and experiencing minimal chronic stress.

But with industrialization, urbanization, and the rise of processed convenience, our health has transformed dramatically. Conventional, modern approaches often contribute to the progression of chronic disease, like putting a simple Band-Aid on a wound that clearly needs stitches. In contrast, a root-cause approach, which targets the factors that contribute to health struggles from the start, has the potential to eliminate or even prevent disease before it ever takes hold:

| Conventional Approach | Root-Cause Approach |
|---|---|
| Medications to mask symptoms | Address the underlying cause |
| Treating disease reactively | Preventing disease proactively |
| Quick fixes | Long-term lifestyle changes |
| Dependence on pharmaceuticals | Empowerment through nutrition & movement |

Chronic disease didn't *appear* overnight. It was built upon, one lifestyle shift at a time. Understanding this evolution, and the root causes, is the first step in reclaiming our health and reversing the damage that modernization has caused our bodies.

## The Standard American Diet (SAD) and Nutritional Deficiencies

**The Problem:** The modern diet is packed with processed foods, refined sugars, and unhealthy fats, leading to systemic inflammation and insulin resistance.

**The Research:** A study in *The Journal of the American Medical Association (JAMA)* found that **60%** of the American diet comes from ultra-processed foods, directly linked to obesity, diabetes, and heart disease.

**The Action Step:** Swap one processed meal this week for a whole, nutrient-dense meal. Try something with fresh vegetables, whole grains, and a free-range or grass-fed organic meat.

## Chronic Stress and the Impact of Cortisol

**The Problem:** Our ancestors experienced short bursts of stress: hunting for food, escaping predators, or surviving harsh weather. Today, stress is chronic and relentless: deadlines, financial worries, social pressures, and digital overload keep our cortisol levels elevated.

**The Research:** Studies published in *Psychoneuroendocrinology* link long-term stress to hypertension, depression, and autoimmune diseases.

**The Action Step:** Take five deep breaths right now: inhale slowly through your nose, hold for a moment, then exhale through your mouth. Deep breathing signals your nervous system to relax, lowers cortisol levels, and reduces stress instantly.

## Sleep Deprivation and Circadian Disruption

**The Problem:** Poor sleep habits disrupt your hormones, impair cognitive function, and lead to a higher risk of metabolic dysfunction.

**The Research:** Research from *Nature Communications* found that sleep deprivation increases inflammation and insulin resistance, setting the stage for developing chronic disease.

**The Action Step:** Turn off screens at least 30 minutes before bed tonight to improve your sleep quality. Disconnect from all blue light from phones, tablets, and TVs to signal to your body that it's time to wind down.

## Toxins and Environmental Pollutants

**The Problem:** We are bombarded daily with harmful chemicals in food, water, household products, and even the air we breathe, all of which disrupt metabolism and hormone function.

**The Research:** Microplastics have been found in human blood, lung tissue, and even placentas: highlighting the pervasive exposure to plastic toxins. Studies like the *U.S. Geological Survey (USGS)* have detected PFAS ("forever chemicals") in tap water across major cities, contributing to liver damage, reproductive issues, and cancer risk.

**The Action Step:** Use a high-quality water filter to minimize exposure to toxins in your drinking water. Consider filtering both drinking and cooking water for maximum protection.

## The Myth of Genetics: Why 90% of Chronic Disease is Within Our Control

Many believe chronic disease is a result of genetic fate, but **epigenetics**, the study of how lifestyle choices influence gene expression, tells a different story, proving that we have more control over our health than we once thought.

**The Research:** The *American Journal of Clinical Nutrition* confirms that **only 10%** of disease risk is genetic; the other **90%** is determined by lifestyle.

**The Reality?** The healthcare system manages symptoms from disease, rather than promote prevention.

**The Action Step:** Choose one small habit today that positively impacts your long-term health tomorrow, and every day after.

## You Have the Power to Heal

I've witnessed firsthand how chronic disease can rob people of their potential, vitality, and joy, but I've also seen journeys of incredible transformation when people fight back against unhealthy triggers. This book's goal is to give you the knowledge, tools, and confidence to acknowledge, inform, and empower your own journey to reclaim your health, no matter where you're starting from.

Chronic disease is not a matter of bad luck; it's the result of repeated lifestyle choices, compounded by a modern world that often promotes sickness. Just as it *developed*, it can be *reversed*. You don't need permission to take control of your health, that decision is yours.

### Next Up

In **Chapter 3**, we'll dive into how metabolic health is the key foundation for preventing and reversing disease, along with secrets and tips to accessing your metabolic health to work *for* you, not against you.

# Chapter 3:
# Metabolic Health: Ignite Your Body's Natural Healing

Did You Know? The Secret to Longevity Lies in Metabolism

**Metabolic dysfunction is responsible for over 85% of chronic diseases, including diabetes, heart disease, and obesity, yet most people don't even realize their metabolism is failing until it's too late.**

At just 38, Amy felt exhausted every day before it even started. She was overweight, constantly fatigued, and prediabetic. Her doctor dismissed it as "bad genetics," but Amy refused to accept that as her fate. She took control: changing her diet, starting strength training, working with a homeopath, and incorporating intermittent fasting. Within six months, she lost 40 pounds, reversed her prediabetes symptoms, and regained her energy. Amy didn't just change her *diet*, she changed her *future*. And you can too.

Think of your metabolism as a fire burning in a furnace. When properly fueled, it burns steadily, providing warmth and energy. But if the fuel is poor-quality, like processed foods, sugar, and a lack of movement, the fire smolders, producing smoke (inflammation) and barely generating heat (energy). Over time, the fire weakens and eventually dies out. To keep your metabolic fire burning strong, you need the right fuel (nutrient-dense foods), proper airflow (movement and exercise), and routine maintenance (quality sleep and stress management). When you take control, you can reignite your fire.

Your metabolism isn't just about burning calories: it's the cornerstone of your overall health. By optimizing it, you can not only prevent chronic disease but, in some cases, even reverse it.

## Why Metabolism Is the Key to Preventing and Reversing Disease

Metabolism is more than just weight loss. It is the process by which your body:

- **Converts food** into usable energy.
- **Repairs and regenerates** cells and tissues.
- **Balances hormones** that affect everything from mood to hunger.
- **Regulates inflammation** and **immune function**.

When your metabolism functions *optimally*, you feel energized, maintain a healthy weight, and keep disease at bay. But when it *slows down*, symptoms like weight gain, fatigue, brain fog, and inflammation take over. This sets the stage for chronic conditions such as diabetes, heart disease, and more. Optimizing your metabolism is key to preventing these health challenges and reclaiming vitality.

## Myths vs. Truths: Your Metabolism

| Myth | Truth |
|---|---|
| Weight gain occurs simply from eating too many calories. | The quality of calories matters more than the quantity because not all calories are processed the same way by the body.<br>• Processed carbs spike insulin and lead to fat storage.<br>• Healthy fats and proteins fuel the body efficiently without blood sugar crashes.<br>• Nutrient timing (when you eat) affects metabolism just as much as what you eat. |
| **Action Step**: Swap one processed carb (e.g., white bread) for a whole food alternative (e.g., sprouted grain bread) today. ||

| A slow metabolism is genetic, and there's nothing you can do about it. | While genetics play a small role, lifestyle choices like diet, exercise, and sleep have a much greater impact on metabolic health. Studies show that strength training, nutrient timing, and optimizing sleep can significantly boost metabolic function. |
|---|---|

**Action Step**: Incorporate strength training (e.g., squats, deadlifts, or push-ups) at least 2-3 times per week to naturally increase muscle mass and metabolic rate.

| Eating small meals throughout the day keeps your metabolism high. | The total amount of food you eat matters more than meal frequency. Research shows that intermittent fasting or spacing meals properly can improve metabolism, insulin sensitivity, and fat burning. |
|---|---|

**Action Step**: Try fasting for 12-14 hours overnight to allow your body to reset and optimize metabolic function.

| Cardio is the best way to boost your metabolism and lose weight. | While cardio benefits heart health, strength training is more effective for increasing metabolism in the long run since muscle burns more calories at rest than fat. Excessive cardio without strength training can actually slow metabolism by breaking down muscle mass. |
|---|---|

**Action Step:** Prioritize resistance training (e.g., bands and weights) over excessive cardio for sustainable fat loss and metabolic health.

## How Metabolic Dysfunction Leads to Chronic Disease

Metabolic dysfunction occurs when your body struggles to efficiently *use energy*, resulting in:

- **Weight gain and obesity**: Excess fat storage due to poor energy utilization.

- Fatigue and sluggishness: Cells fail to produce enough energy for the body to function.

- Brain fog and memory loss: Blood sugar imbalances impair cognitive function.

- Inflammation and pain: Persistent low-grade inflammation harms tissue and speeds up aging.

**This dysfunction doesn't happen *overnight*;** it is the result of years of poor dietary choices, sedentary habits, stress, and lack of restorative sleep.

The healthcare industry promotes metabolic dysfunction. Rather than addressing the root causes of diseases like diabetes and obesity, it prioritizes medications that merely "manage" symptoms, turning patients into lifelong customers instead of offering real solutions:

| Conventional Approach | Root-Cause Approach |
|---|---|
| Prescribes medications to lower blood sugar | Uses diet and movement to reverse insulin resistance |
| Treats obesity with weight loss drugs | Heals metabolism through proper nutrition and strength training |
| Recommends calorie restriction and low-fat diets | Encourages whole, nutrient dense foods and fasting practices |

**Action Step:** Identify **one** daily habit that might be harming your metabolism (e.g., skipping meals or sitting for long hours with no breaks) and replace it with a **healthier alternative** (e.g., intentional intermittent fasting or a 30-minute walk).

# The Three Warnings of Metabolic Health

Metabolic health has three key warnings: improper insulin balance, uncontrolled inflammatory responses, and mismanaging your gut health.

By optimizing these three areas, and getting ahead of any lingering or future issues, you can enhance energy levels, maintain a healthy weight, and prevent chronic disease.

## Insulin Resistance: The Hidden Epidemic

Insulin is a crucial hormone that regulates blood sugar levels. However, excessive consumption of refined carbohydrates and sugars can overwhelm this system, causing cells to become resistant to insulin. This insulin resistance leads to:

- **Chronically high blood sugar levels:** This could increase the risk of type 2 diabetes.

- **Increased fat storage, particularly around the abdomen**: Excess sugar is converted into fat instead of being used for energy.

- **Higher risk of serious health conditions:** Including diabetes, heart disease, and neurodegeneration.

**Action Step:** Try **reducing added sugars** (e.g., sweetened coffee, flavored yogurts) for a week and observe the difference in energy and hunger levels.

## Chronic Inflammation: The Silent Saboteur

Inflammation is the body's natural defense mechanism against injury or infection. However, when inflammation becomes chronic, it fuels conditions like diabetes, heart disease, Dementia, Alzheimer's, and autoimmune disorders to develop. Some key contributors to chronic inflammation include:

- **Ultra-processed foods** which are high in sugar and seed oils.
- **Poor sleep and chronic stress** which raises cortisol levels and disrupts the body's ability to regulate inflammation.
- **Lack of physical activity** which reduces the body's detoxification and circulation abilities.

**Action Step:** Add **one anti-inflammatory food** (e.g., turmeric, leafy greens, olive oil) to your meals today.

# Gut Health: The Foundation of Metabolism

Your gut microbiome plays a crucial role in digestion, metabolism, immune function, and even weight regulation. When gut bacteria are out of balance due to a poor diet lacking fiber and healthy fats, it can lead to:

- **Poor nutrient absorption**: A weakened gut lining makes it harder to absorb essential vitamins and minerals.

- **Increased fat storage and cravings**: An imbalance in gut bacteria can trigger sugar cravings, leading to weight gain.

- **Weakened immune function**: Unhealthy gut bacteria can increase susceptibility to infections and chronic disease.

**Action Step:** Eat a **fiber-rich meal** today (e.g., beans, flaxseeds, berries) to feed your good gut bacteria.

A sluggish metabolism can't be fixed by starving yourself. Instead, focus on key strategies that support metabolic health, allowing you to optimize your metabolism without extreme dieting or deprivation. These strategies include:

- **Strength training:** Building muscle increases your metabolic rate.

- **Intermittent fasting:** Short periods of fasting improve insulin sensitivity and fat burning.

- **Whole foods diet:** Cutting out processed foods and focusing on protein, healthy fats, and fiber fuels metabolic efficiency.

- **Quality sleep and stress management:** Regulating stress and prioritizing rest helps balance hormones that control metabolism.

**Action Step:** Start **moving for 10 minutes after each meal** to regulate blood sugar levels and improve metabolism.

# Your 30-Day Action Plan: Metabolic Reset

Kickstarting your metabolism will improve your overall health. Don't feel overwhelmed. Focus on implementing simple yet powerful changes each week that will add up to metabolic optimization. Here's a straightforward, accessible plan to follow:

**WEEK 1: Reset Your Diet**

- Swap out processed foods for whole, nutrient-dense alternatives.
- Drink more water and cut back on sugary drinks.

**WEEK 2: Move Daily**

- Walk for 30 minutes per day, especially after meals.
- Add two days of strength training to your week.

**WEEK 3: Optimize Sleep & Stress**

- Set a consistent sleep schedule to follow every night.
- Practice deep breathing or meditation to manage stress.

**WEEK 4: Reduce Toxins & Improve Gut Health**

- Eat more fiber-rich foods and fermented foods (e.g., kimchi, yogurt).

- Use a high-quality water filter to limit toxin exposure.

I've seen too many people struggle, believing their metabolism is broken or their health is out of their control. But the truth is, you're not stuck; your body is designed to heal.

By taking small, consistent steps today, your future can be radically different. Your energy, longevity, and ability to prevent disease are within your power. Don't let anyone tell you otherwise.

**Next Up**

In **Chapter 4**, we'll explore how **food acts as medicine**, shaping your metabolism and overall well-being.

# PART II:
# Daily Choices That Heal – Your Path to A Disease-Free Life

# Chapter 4:
## Food as Medicine: Eat to Reverse Disease

Did You Know? Every Bite You Take is Either Fighting Disease or Feeding It

**Over 60% of the American diet consists of ultra-processed foods, leading to skyrocketing rates of obesity, diabetes, and heart disease. The right nutrition can prevent and even reverse these conditions.**

Imagine being diagnosed with an incurable autoimmune disease at just 35 years old. That was Emma's reality. Doctors told her she would need lifelong medication with serious side effects. Determined to find another solution, she turned to food as medicine.

By eliminating processed foods, focusing on anti-inflammatory nutrition, and healing her gut, Emma transformed her health. Within a year, her symptoms disappeared, and she no longer needed medication. Her doctor called it a "miracle," but it wasn't, it was *the power of food.*

The food you consume daily directly influences your genes, metabolism, and immune function. This is your **call to action**: your plate can be your greatest defense against disease or your biggest liability. The choice is yours.

**Think of your body like a computer.** The software (your DNA) is designed to function optimally when provided with the right inputs (nutrients). But if you download a virus (processed foods, sugar, inflammatory oils), the system begins to malfunction, leading to disease. The good news? You can rewrite your programming at any time by changing what you eat, like downloading your very own antivirus software.

## The Hidden Reality: Understanding the System Behind Poor Nutrition and Chronic Disease

Many people are unaware that the systems influencing our health, especially food and healthcare, may not always prioritize long-term wellness. Highly processed foods, often marketed as convenient or even healthy, are widely consumed despite their link to lifestyle-related diseases like diabetes, heart disease, and obesity. At the same time, the standard medical model often focuses on managing these conditions with medications, rather than addressing the root causes through nutrition.

This creates a cycle that can be difficult to escape without awareness and effort. That's why it's so important to stay informed and take an active role in your health. By exploring functional nutrition and preventative strategies, individuals can begin to shift from dependency on the system to true healing and vitality.

| Conventional Approach | Root-Cause Approach |
|---|---|
| Medications to control symptoms | Whole foods to reverse disease |
| Prescribed statins for high cholesterol | Eliminating processed foods to restore heart health |
| Medications to manage and control blood sugar levels | Cutting sugar and improving insulin sensitivity |
| Treating obesity with weight-loss pills | Using nutrition to regulate metabolism |

## Myths vs. Truths About Food as Medicine

| Myth | Truth |
|---|---|
| Eating fat makes you fat. | Healthy fats like avocados, olive oil, and nuts help regulate metabolism, balance hormones, and reduce inflammation. It's the |

| | overconsumption of processed sugars and refined carbohydrates that lead to weight gain and disease. |
|---|---|
| **Action Step:** Swap out processed, high-carb snacks for healthy fats like almonds or avocado slices to help improve satiety and metabolism. ||

| | |
|---|---|
| All calories are equal. | The quality of calories matters more than the quantity. For example, 100 calories from soda affects your body differently than 100 calories from broccoli. Processed foods spike insulin and inflammation, while whole foods nourish and heal. |
| **Action Step:** Focus on your intake of nutrient-dense foods rather than counting calories; opt for whole, unprocessed options at every meal. ||

| | |
|---|---|
| You need dairy for strong bones. | While dairy does contain calcium, many plant-based sources like leafy greens, almonds, and sesame seeds provide just as much (if not more) bioavailable calcium *without* inflammation-causing additives. |
| **Action Step:** Try swapping out dairy for a plant-based calcium source, such as kale, chia seeds, or tahini. Nut-based milks are also a healthier option to regular dairy products. ||

# The Anti-Inflammatory Diet: What to Eat & What to Avoid

Chronic inflammation is at the root of nearly all major diseases, including heart disease, diabetes, and autoimmune disorders. The foods you eat either help calm and reduce inflammation or fuel it, making dietary choices a powerful tool for disease prevention. Anti-inflammatory foods like leafy greens, fatty fish, turmeric, and berries help calm the immune system and promote healing.

On the other hand, processed foods, refined sugars, and industrial seed oils trigger chronic inflammation, increasing the risk of illness. Understanding which foods support or harm your body is crucial for long-term health.

## What to Eat: Healing, Nutrient-Dense Foods

**Vegetables & Fruits**: Leafy greens, cruciferous veggies, berries, citrus fruits, and avocados are packed with antioxidants and fiber.

**Healthy Fats**: Omega-3 fatty acids from wild-caught fish, flaxseeds, and walnuts reduce inflammation.

**Lean Proteins**: Grass-fed meats, pasture-raised eggs, and plant-based proteins support muscle and metabolic function.

**Whole Grains**: Quinoa, brown rice, millet, and oats stabilize blood sugar and provide essential nutrients.

**Herbs & Spices**: Turmeric, ginger, garlic, and cinnamon offer powerful anti-inflammatory benefits.

## What to Avoid: Inflammatory, Disease-Promoting Foods

**Processed Foods**: Packaged snacks, refined grains, and fast food are filled with preservatives and trans fats.

**Refined Sugar**: High sugar (white, brown, high fructose corn syrup) intake spikes insulin, fuels inflammation, and promotes weight gain.

**Industrial Seed Oils**: Corn, soybean, and canola oils are loaded with omega-6s that drive inflammation.

**Dairy & Gluten**: Many people have hidden sensitivities (lactose intolerance and celiacs disease) that trigger gut inflammation when ingesting too much dairy and gluten products, including milk, eggs, cheese, wheat, barley, and rye.

**Action Step:** Swap one inflammatory food for a healing food today (e.g., replace sugar-laden cereal with a smoothie packed with greens and berries).

## The Hidden Regulator: The Endocannabinoid System & Inflammation Control

The **Endocannabinoid System (ECS)** is the body's built-in, natural regulatory network that helps maintain balance (homeostasis) by controlling inflammation, immune response, pain, mood, and metabolism at the cellular level. It plays a crucial role in reducing chronic inflammation. By supporting the ECS through nutrition, stress management, and lifestyle choices, you can enhance its ability to promote healing and reverse chronic disease naturally.

### How to Activate the ECS for Healing

**Eat more healthy fats:** For example, omega-3s from wild fish and various seeds enhance ECS function.

**Use plant-based cannabinoids:** CBD and other phytocannabinoids, cannabinoids that occur naturally in the cannabis plant, support ECS regulation. The science is evolving on CBD, and the information presented should not be interpreted as conclusive or as a replacement for professional medical guidance.

**Manage stress & sleep well**: Chronic stress weakens ECS function and increases inflammation, while irregular sleep creates an imbalance in the ECS system.

**Action Step:** Add one omega-3-rich food to your diet today (e.g., walnuts, flaxseeds, or salmon).

## How Sugar & Processed Foods Fuel Disease

Scientific research consistently confirms that excess sugar and processed foods are directly linked to obesity, diabetes, and heart disease by driving insulin resistance, chronic inflammation, and metabolic dysfunction. The first step to overcoming a sugar craving is to fully understand and accept the harm it's causing on a daily basis:

### How Sugar Harms Your Health

**Increases insulin resistance** leading to diabetes and metabolic dysfunction.
**Feeds harmful gut bacteria**, causing digestive issues and immune dysfunction.
**Disrupts hormones that regulate hunger**, leading to overeating and weight gain.

**Action Step:** Reduce added sugar intake for one week and track how you feel. Track changes in energy levels, cravings, mood, digestion, and sleep quality.

## The Best Foods for Healing & Energy

Healthy foods have the power to *reset* your body's internal systems, and you have the power to choose the healthy over the unhealthy options.

Here's a brief beginners guide on how to start eating to heal:

### For Reducing Inflammation:

- **Fatty fish:** salmon, sardines, mackerel
- **Leafy greens**: spinach, kale, Swiss chard
- **Nuts & seeds**: almonds, walnuts, flaxseeds

### For Balancing Hormones:

- **Cruciferous veggies**: broccoli, Brussels sprouts, cauliflower
- **Avocados**: rich in healthy fats and fiber
- **Maca root**: supports adrenal health

**For Boosting Energy:**

- **Complex carbs**: sweet potatoes, quinoa, lentils

- **High-quality proteins**: grass-fed beef, organic poultry

- **Hydrating foods**: cucumber, watermelon, coconut water

**Action Step:** Add one energy-boosting food to your next meal.

## 1-Day Healing Meal Plan & Simple Recipes

Once you have your healthy ingredients, you can start incorporating them into your daily meals. Below is a sample 1-day meal plan along with a quick recipe to help you kickstart your healthier habits:

**Sample Meal Plan:**

- **Breakfast:** Scrambled eggs with spinach & avocado, side of berries.

- **Lunch:** Grilled salmon with quinoa & roasted vegetables.

- **Snack:** Handful of walnuts & a green smoothie.

- **Dinner:** Turmeric-spiced chicken with sautéed kale & sweet potato mash.

## Quick Recipe: Anti-Inflammatory Turmeric Smoothie:

| Ingredients: | Instructions: |
|---|---|
| <ul><li>1 cup unsweetened almond milk</li><li>1 banana</li><li>½ tsp turmeric</li><li>½ tsp cinnamon</li><li>1 tbsp flax seeds</li><li>1 handful spinach</li><li>Ice cubes (optional)</li></ul> | Blend all ingredients until smooth. Enjoy as a refreshing, anti-inflammatory boost. |

# Your 30-Day Action Plan: Nutrition Reset

Changing what we eat, how we shop for groceries, and how we prepare food can feel like a big undertaking. However, by making small, step-by-step changes over time, you can gradually transform your eating habits to promote overall health. Here's a simple and accessible plan for your first month:

**WEEK 1: Stock Your Kitchen**

- Keep fresh vegetables, fruits, healthy fats, & quality proteins on hand.

**WEEK 2: Eliminate Processed Foods & Sugar**

- Read labels & avoid artificial ingredients like sweeteners, colors, and preservatives.

**WEEK 3: Cook More at Home**

- Preparing meals, even meal prepping, lets you control ingredients & maximize nutrition.

## WEEK 4: Hydrate & Eat Mindfully

- Drink clean, filtered water & slow down at meals. Chewing slowly and focusing on food intake can make a huge difference.

Every meal is a chance to **fight disease or fuel it**.

The choice is yours. I've seen too many people struggle with chronic conditions that could have been prevented, or even reversed, with the right nutrition. When you start nourishing your body with real, whole foods, you'll be amazed at how quickly your energy returns, inflammation subsides, and your symptoms fade. You deserve to thrive, not just survive.

## Next Up

In **Chapter 5**, we'll explore the power of movement and how exercise and movement overall is essential for healing and longevity.

# Chapter 5:
## Movement Matters: Heal Your Body Through Exercise

## Did You Know? Sitting Too Much Can Be as Bad as Smoking

**Physical inactivity is now one of the leading causes of preventable deaths worldwide, linked to similar deaths than smoking, according to The Lancet.**

What if, at 45, you were told your body was aging faster than someone 20 years *older*, all because you weren't moving enough? That was Tom's reality. Years of sitting at a desk, avoiding exercise, and staying inactive took a toll, leading to severe joint pain, metabolic syndrome, and prediabetes. His doctor's advice was clear: exercise could do more for him than any medication. Determined to turn things around, Tom committed to daily walks and strength training twice a week. Six months later, his blood sugar normalized, his joint pain disappeared, and he felt more energized than he had in years.

Tom didn't just start moving; he reclaimed his life.

Movement is the closest thing to a miracle drug. Your body is ready: *are you?*

Imagine a river that once flowed freely, nourishing everything in its path. Now picture that river being blocked: water grows stagnant, algae spreads, and life begins to fade.

The same happens to our bodies when we stop moving. Stagnation leads to sluggish circulation, toxin buildup, and a slowing metabolism. But when you restore movement, you restore vitality: blood flows, toxins are flushed, and your body reawakens. Movement isn't just activity; it's the key to keeping life flowing within you.

## Why Movement Isn't Always Prioritized in Modern Healthcare

In today's fast-paced world, physical activity is often overlooked, despite its well-documented benefits for preventing and managing chronic disease. This may be due in part to the way our systems are structured. Pharmaceutical solutions are more commonly emphasized in medical training than lifestyle-based interventions. At the same time, much of modern marketing encourages sedentary habits, from fast food convenience to screen-heavy entertainment and desk-bound work environments.

While medications and technology have their place, individuals facing chronic health challenges deserve a more holistic approach. Being informed and proactive, incorporating movement, nutrition, and other integrative strategies, can be a powerful step toward lasting health and vitality.

| Conventional Approach | Root-Cause Approach |
|---|---|
| Prescribes medication for high blood pressure | Uses daily movement to naturally lower blood pressure |
| Treats obesity with weight-loss drugs | Encourages strength training to build muscle and burn fat naturally |
| Recommends surgeries for joint pain | Improves mobility with exercise and functional movement |

## The Science of Movement & Longevity

Extensive scientific research confirms that regular movement is one of the most powerful tools for reversing chronic diseases such as heart diseases and extending your lifespan. A landmark study from *Harvard Medical School* found that 150 minutes of moderate-intensity exercise per week reduces the risk of early death by 31%. Some other findings that support this claim include:

**Boosts mitochondrial function**: This causes your body's energy factories to work better, slowing aging in the process.

**Reduces inflammation**: Exercise regulates inflammatory markers which protect against disease.

**Enhances brain function**: Regular movement increases blood flow to the brain which reduces dementia risk.

**Improves hormonal balance**: Movement regulates insulin, cortisol, and other key hormones that affect your metabolism.

**Action Step:** Try setting a timer to move every hour, even if it's just a quick stretch.

## Myths vs. Truths About Exercise

| Myth | Truth |
|---|---|
| You need to do long, intense workouts every day to see results. | Short, consistent workouts are more effective for long-term health than sporadic, extreme exercise. Even 10-minute daily walks can significantly reduce disease risk and improve longevity. |
| **Action Step:** Aim for at least 10-15 minutes of movement every day, whether it's walking, stretching, or strength training. ||

| Cardio is the best way to lose weight. | Strength training builds muscle, which increases metabolism and burns fat even at rest. While cardio is great for heart health, lifting weights is more effective for long-term fat loss and metabolic health. |
| --- | --- |
| **Action Step:** Incorporate 2-to-3 strength training sessions per week to maintain muscle mass and boost your metabolism. | |

| If you're not sweating, you're not working hard enough. | Not all beneficial movement requires sweating. Yoga, stretching, and walking improve flexibility, reduce stress, and boost recovery all without causing excessive sweating in most cases. |
| --- | --- |
| **Action Step:** Try low-impact exercises, like yoga, pilates or tai chi, once a week to improve mobility and reduce stress. | |

## The Best Types of Exercise for Healing & Longevity

The best types of exercise for healing and longevity focus on improving mobility, strength, and cardiovascular health while reducing inflammation and stress. Strength training, high-intensity interval training, and flexibility training are all very beneficial examples.

A well-rounded approach that includes a mix of these exercises promotes healing, prevents chronic disease, and supports a longer, healthier life.

**Strength Training: The Metabolism Booster:**

- Builds **lean muscle**, increasing metabolic rate.
- Enhances **bone density**, reducing osteoporosis risk.
- Lowers **blood sugar**, reversing insulin resistance.

**Try This:** Two or three strength sessions per week (bodyweight exercises, resistance bands, or lifting weights).

**High-Intensity Interval Training (HIIT): The Fat-Burning Accelerator:**

- Alternates **short bursts** of intense movement with rest.
- Proven to **reverse** metabolic syndrome and improve cardiovascular health.

**Try This:** 20-minute HIIT session including sprinting, jumping jacks, or cycling.

**Yoga & Tai Chi: The Mind-Body Connection:**

- Enhances **flexibility, balance,** and **mental well-being**.

- Lowers **cortisol levels**, reducing stress and inflammation.

**Try This:** 15-30 minutes of yoga or tai chi daily for stress and mobility.

## How Walking Alone Can Reverse Disease

You don't need an expensive gym membership to transform your health. Walking is one of the simplest and most effective ways to prevent and even reverse disease. A study from *Harvard Medical School* found that walking 7,000 to 10,000 steps per day can cut the risk of early death by 50%.

**Walking Benefits:**

- Reduces heart disease risk by **30%**.
- Lowers blood pressure & improves cholesterol levels.
- Boosts mood & cognitive function.

**Action Step:** Take a 10-minute walk after meals to aid digestion & blood sugar control.

## Practical Tips to Make Movement a Habit

Here are a few easy, accessible tips to incorporate daily that will get you up & moving:

1. **Move Every Hour**: Set a reminder to stand up and stretch.
2. **Take the Stairs**: Skip the elevator when possible.
3. **Play More**: Dance, swim, play a sport: make movement fun!
4. **Use a Standing Desk**: Reduce prolonged sitting at work.
5. **Set a Daily Step Goal**: Track daily steps with a smartwatch or app.

**Action Step:** Choose and commit to **one** of these daily habits to incorporate into your lifestyle in order to increase your movement.

# Your 30-Day Action Plan: Movement Reset

Exercise isn't about punishment or aesthetics: it's about reclaiming your vitality. By making movement a daily habit, you unlock your body's natural ability to heal, regenerate, and thrive. You don't have to overhaul your life overnight. Start small, stay consistent, and watch as your body rewards you with more energy, strength, and resilience than you ever thought possible.

Here's a step-by-step, week-by-week plan to help you incorporate movement into your life during your first month:

**WEEK 1: Start Small**

- Move for **5 minutes every hour**.
- **Walk after meals** to improve metabolism.

**WEEK 2: Add Strength**

- Add **2 to 3 days of bodyweight or resistance training** per week.
- Focus on **compound movements** (squats, push-ups).

**WEEK 3: Increase Intensity**

- **Add short HIIT sessions** (jump rope, sprints).

- Challenge yourself with **longer walks or hikes.**

**WEEK 4: Mind-Body Balance**

- Try adding **yoga, tai chi,** or **breathwork** into your routine to reduce stress.

- Mix up movement styles to keep it **enjoyable.**

You don't have to wait for *permission* to move. Your body was designed to move, and movement is the key to reversing chronic disease. I've seen far too many people suffer from conditions that could have been prevented simply by staying active. Movement is not a punishment; it's a gift. It's not about running marathons or lifting heavy weights; it's about reclaiming your ability to thrive.

### Next Up

In **Chapter 6**, we'll explore the role and importance of sleep & stress management in reversing chronic disease.

# Chapter 6:

## Sleep and Stress: The Hidden Threats Sabotaging Your Health

Did You Know? Chronic Stress and Poor Sleep Are as Harmful as a Bad Diet

**Sleep deprivation and chronic stress increase the risk of heart disease, diabetes, and early death as much as smoking and poor diet. A single night of bad sleep can spike cortisol, disrupt insulin, and trigger inflammation, making it one of the most overlooked factors in chronic disease.**

Imagine being a high-performing executive, surviving on five hours of sleep, fueled by coffee, and believing rest is a sign of weakness. That was Lisa's reality, until her body hit rock bottom. At 48, she developed severe adrenal fatigue, weight gain, and chronic inflammation. No medication worked until she made one *crucial* change: prioritizing sleep and reducing her stress. Within six months, Lisa regained her energy, improved her insulin resistance, and finally felt like herself again.

This is your wake-up call: sleep and stress have a bigger impact on your health than you realize. Just like a phone needs to recharge, so does your body. If you want to *heal*, start by taking control of your rest and stress levels.

Imagine your body as a high-performance vehicle, you wouldn't expect it to run smoothly without proper fuel and regular maintenance. Yet, many of us push our bodies to the limit, running on little sleep and constant stress. Just as an engine overheats when overworked, your body breaks down when deprived of rest and recovery. To function at your best, you must prioritize restoration just as much as action.

Chronic stress and sleep deprivation **fuel** the pharmaceutical industry much like food and a sedentary lifestyle do. Some examples of how include:

- Insomnia? Here's a **sleeping pill.**
- Anxiety? Here's an **antidepressant.**
- High blood pressure? Here's a **lifetime of medication.**

Instead of addressing the root cause, poor sleep, high stress, and lifestyle factors, conventional medicine relies on endless prescriptions.

| Conventional Approach | Root-Cause Approach |
|---|---|
| Sleeping pills for insomnia | Natural sleep hygiene practices |
| Antidepressants for anxiety | Stress-reducing lifestyle habits |
| Caffeine to fight fatigue | Prioritizing deep, restorative sleep |
| Treating high cortisol with medications | Using meditation, breathwork, and nature to regulate stress |

**The reality?** Sleep challenges have fueled a $40 billion pharmaceutical market, highlighting how solutions often focus on symptom relief rather than addressing the root causes of fatigue. That's why being informed and exploring holistic approaches to rest and recovery is so important.

## How Stress Fuels Chronic Disease (And How to Stop It)

Stress isn't *inherently* bad. In small doses, it can sharpen focus and build resilience. But when stress becomes chronic, it's like running a car engine on overdrive for too long. It eventually overheats and breaks down.

Your body needs periods of rest and recovery to function at its best.

## The Consequences of Chronic Stress:

**Chronic Inflammation**: A driver of heart disease, diabetes, and autoimmune disorders.

**Hormonal Imbalances**: Elevated cortisol levels lead to weight gain, insomnia, and the development of mood disorders.

**Weakened Immunity**: Stress suppresses the immune system, making you more susceptible to illness.

## Breaking the Stress Cycle

Here are some easy, accessible ways to begin tackling stress in order to break the cycle:

- **Breathe with intention**: Try **box breathing** (inhale for 4 seconds, hold for 4, exhale for 4) to instantly reduce stress in the moment.

- **Reconnect with nature**: Studies show that spending time in green spaces lowers cortisol and improves your mood.

- **Practice gratitude**: A daily gratitude journal rewires the brain to focus on positive experiences.

**Action Step:** Take **5 minutes** today to practice deep breathing or gratitude journaling.

## Myths vs. Truths About Sleep & Stress

| Myth | Truth |
|---|---|
| You can function just fine on 4 to 5 hours of sleep a night. | Less than **1%** of the population has a rare genetic mutation allowing them to function well on limited sleep. For everyone else, lack of sleep damages memory, metabolism, and immunity. |
| **Action Step:** Prioritize 7 to 9 hours of high-quality sleep each night. ||

| Stress only affects you mentally. | Stress creates physical damage in the body, elevating cortisol, increasing inflammation, and worsening chronic disease. Even if you don't feel anxious, stress could still be harming your metabolism and immune system. |
|---|---|
| **Action Step:** Implement a daily relaxation practice, such as deep breathing, mindfulness, or time in nature. ||

| If you can't fall asleep, just stay in bed until you eventually do. | Lying awake in bed conditions your brain to associate your bed with restlessness. If you can't fall asleep after 20 minutes, get up, do a relaxing activity, and return to bed when you feel tired. |
| --- | --- |

**Action Step:** Develop a bedtime wind-down routine with dim lighting, deep breathing, and no screens 30 minutes before sleep.

# The Underestimated Power of Sleep in Healing the Body

We live in a society that glorifies hustle and late-night productivity, but science paints a different picture. Sleep is the body's ultimate reset button, essential for cellular repair, memory consolidation, and hormone balance. Prioritizing rest isn't a luxury: it's a necessity for optimal health and performance. A body deprived of sleep is a body in trouble.

**The Dangers of Sleep Deprivation:**

- **Increases toxic protein buildup in the brain**, raising the risk of Alzheimer's (*Science Advances*).

- **Alters hunger hormones**, leading to increased appetite and weight gain.

- **Impairs insulin sensitivity**, contributing to diabetes and cardiovascular disease.

## Optimizing Sleep for Better Health

A number of small lifestyle changes can improve your sleep habits and contribute to better overall health. A few of these include:

- **Keep a Consistent Sleep Schedule**: Going to bed and waking up at the same time stabilizes circadian rhythms.

- **Create a Sleep-Friendly Environment**: Keep your bedroom cool (65°F), dark, and free from screens.

- **Limit Stimulants**: Avoid caffeine and blue light exposure at least 2 hours before bed.

**Action Step:** Set a bedtime alarm as a reminder to start winding down at least 2 hours before you plan to go to sleep.

# Natural Ways to Improve Sleep & Manage Stress

Harnessing **natural remedies** can significantly improve sleep quality and stress resilience, without relying on a prescribed sleeping aid. Some of these include:

- **Magnesium Supplementation**: Promotes relaxation by regulating neurotransmitters.

- **Adaptogenic Herbs (Ashwagandha, Rhodiola)**: Helps modulate cortisol levels, reducing stress-induced fatigue.

- **Mindfulness Meditation**: *Harvard Medical School* research shows mindfulness practice enhances sleep and reduces stress by calming the amygdala (the brain's fear center).

**Action Step:** Try magnesium or a calming herbal tea before bed.

*Any nutritional or supplement recommendations are intended to support general wellness and are not meant to diagnose, treat, or prevent any disease. Consult your healthcare provider before starting any diet or supplement program.

# The Endocannabinoid System & Sleep Regulation

Your **Endocannabinoid System (ECS)** is a complex network of receptors, enzymes, and endocannabinoids that helps regulate several physiological processes, including sleep. It plays a crucial role in promoting deep, restorative sleep by balancing neurotransmitter activity and reducing stress-induced wakefulness. By maintaining this balance, the ECS supports a more *restful* and *consistent* sleep cycle, essential for overall health and well-being.

**How Cannabinoids Support Sleep:**

- **CBD nourishes the ECS**, helping to calm the nervous system and reduce nighttime anxiety.
- Unlike pharmaceutical sleep aids, cannabinoids **naturally support the body's ability to fall asleep and stay asleep.**

**Action Step:** Consider a natural ECS-supporting supplement for deeper sleep like CBD.

*Some topics discussed in this book reflect emerging areas of research. The science is evolving, and the information presented should not be interpreted as conclusive or as a replacement for professional medical guidance.

# The Mind-Body Connection: How Mindset Affects Your Biology

Your thoughts aren't just abstract; they directly impact your biology. A *PNAS (Proceedings of the National Academy of Sciences)* study found that people with a strong sense of purpose had *lower* inflammation and *longer* lifespans.

**Reframing Your Mindset for Health:**

- **Visualize Healing**: Guided imagery like BrainTap, a wearable device that optimizes your brain's potential using sessions of guided brainwave exercises, helps program the brain for recovery and optimum health.

- **Adopt a Growth Mindset**: Shift your perspective in order to view challenges as opportunities, not obstacles.

- **Surround Yourself with Positivity**: Engage with uplifting, like-minded communities that inspire and support your growth.

**Action Step:** Write **one** positive affirmation about your health today in a journal, if it feels good, repeat the step the next day.

# Your 30-Day Action Plan: Sleep & Stress Reset

Sleep and stress management aren't just luxuries: they're *essential* for reversing chronic disease. By prioritizing rest, relaxation, and mindset shifts, you empower your body to heal, regenerate, and thrive. When you start treating sleep as a non-negotiable, everything else in your life will improve: your mood, your energy, and your health. Here's a step-by-step, week-by-week plan to help you improve your sleep & stress for the first month:

## WEEK 1: Prioritize Sleep

- Set a **consistent bedtime** (even on weekends).
- Reduce **caffeine and screen time** in the evening.

## WEEK 2: Implement Stress Breaks

- Take **5-minute mindfulness breaks** throughout the day.
- Spend **10+ minutes outside daily**.

## WEEK 3: Optimize Your Sleep Environment

- Lower bedroom temperature to **65°F**.
- Use **blackout curtains and white noise machines** if needed.

**WEEK 4: Build Resilience**

- Practice **deep breathing or meditation before bed**.

- Write down **3 things you're grateful for** each night.

**Action Step:** Choose **one habit** from the list above and start today.

You don't have to wait for permission to rest. Your body *needs* sleep just as much as it needs food and movement. I've seen how lack of sleep and chronic stress silently destroy people's health. You deserve to rest, you deserve peace. Your body is designed to heal itself, but only if you allow it the time to do so.

## Next Up

In **Chapter 7**, we'll explore the toxic burden of modern living and how to begin detoxifying your body on your journey to optimal health.

# Chapter 7:

# Detox Your Life: Free Your Body from Harmful Toxins

## Did You Know? Your Environment Could Be Making You Sick

**A study from the Environmental Working Group found that the average newborn baby has over 200 industrial chemicals in their umbilical cord blood at birth. This means that before we even take our first breath, we are already exposed to toxins that can disrupt hormones, metabolism, and brain function.**

Amy, a 38-year-old mother of two, struggled with constant fatigue, stubborn weight gain, and brain fog. Despite trying diet and exercise, she saw little improvement. It wasn't until she eliminated toxins from her home, switched to organic foods, and started filtering her water that her body finally *began to heal*. Within three months, Amy regained her energy, lost weight naturally, and experienced improved mental clarity. Your body wants to heal; it just sometimes needs you to *remove* the obstacles standing in its way.

Think of your body as a house with open windows. Fresh air flows in, sunlight brightens the space, and everything feels clean and vibrant. But over time, if you stop cleaning, let clutter pile up, and allow toxic fumes from chemicals to linger, the air becomes stale, mold forms in the corners, and the once-refreshing space turns *suffocating*. Your body works in the same way. Every day, you're exposed to toxins, from the food you eat, the air you breathe, and even the stress you carry.

When these toxins build up without being cleared out, your system becomes sluggish, inflammation increases, and your body struggles to perform at its best. Detoxing is like opening the windows, clearing out the clutter, and restoring your body's natural ability to *thrive*. It's time to declutter your system, clear out the toxins, and create a fresh, clean environment where your health can flourish.

*Will you open the windows and let the healing begin?*

**The reality?** Much of the pharmaceutical industry's success is tied to managing chronic conditions. While medications can be life-saving and necessary, the broader system often focuses on symptom relief rather than root-cause healing, such as addressing environmental stressors, lifestyle factors, or nutritional imbalances.

- **High blood pressure?** Often met with a prescription.

- **Hormonal imbalance?** Frequently treated with synthetic hormones.
- **Chronic fatigue?** Commonly countered with caffeine or stimulants.

This is why it's essential to be informed and explore holistic options that support true healing, not just short-term relief.

| Conventional Approach | Root-Cause Approach |
|---|---|
| Medication for hormone imbalances | Removing endocrine disruptors (plastics, pesticides) |
| Antacids for acid reflux | Improving gut health by eliminating processed foods |
| Sleeping pills for insomnia | Reducing blue light and stress exposure before bed |
| Painkillers for inflammation | Supporting detox pathways with nutrition & hydration |

**What's missing?** Removing the toxins causing these problems in the first place.

# Myths vs. Truths About Detoxing

| Myth | Truth |
|---|---|
| The body detoxes itself, so you don't need to do anything. | While the liver and kidneys do naturally detoxify the body, modern exposure to toxins overwhelms these systems. Supporting detox pathways with the right foods, hydration, and lifestyle changes is essential. |
| **Action Step:** Drink at least 8 cups of filtered water daily and consume cruciferous vegetables (like broccoli and Brussels sprouts) to enhance liver detox. ||

| Myth | Truth |
|---|---|
| Detoxing means doing extreme juice cleanses. | Fasting and cleanses can help, but long-term detoxification comes from sustainable daily habits like eating whole foods, avoiding toxins, and staying hydrated. |
| **Action Step:** Replace one processed meal a day with a nutrient-dense, whole-food meal. ||

| Myth | Truth |
|---|---|
| Toxins only come from pollution and food. | Toxins are everywhere: household cleaners, skincare products, plastics, and even in tap water. Everyday exposure adds up and impacts metabolism, immunity, and brain function. |

## The Hidden Chemicals in Food, Water, and Household Products That Disrupt Health

Toxins are everywhere; often hidden in plain sight. They can be found in processed foods, plastics, personal care products, and even tap water. Some of the most concerning toxins include:

- **Pesticides & Herbicides**: Found in conventionally grown produce, linked to hormone disruption and cancer.
- **Heavy Metals (Lead, Mercury, Arsenic)**: Found in contaminated water, seafood, and old pipes, linked to neurological and metabolic disorders.
- **Endocrine Disruptors**: Found in plastics, cosmetics, and cleaning products, mimic hormones and contribute to weight gain, thyroid issues, and fertility problems.

*A Journal of Clinical Endocrinology & Metabolism* study found that exposure to endocrine-disrupting chemicals is linked to **obesity, metabolic disorders, and even early puberty in children**. These toxins interfere with hormonal balance and chronic inflammation, setting the stage for disease in younger generations.

# How Environmental Toxins Contribute to Hormonal Imbalance and Metabolic Dysfunction

Your body's hormonal system is like a finely tuned orchestra, carefully regulating metabolism, mood, and overall health. But environmental toxins act like out-of-tune instruments, throwing off the balance and disrupting the harmony, leading to imbalances that can affect your well-being.

**How Toxins Impact Your Health:**

- **Weight Gain & Insulin Resistance**: **BPA** (found in plastics) mimics estrogen, promoting fat storage and diabetes risk.

- **Thyroid Dysfunction**: **Fluoride**, commonly found in tap water, suppresses thyroid function, leading to fatigue and weight gain.

- **Brain Fog & Neurological Issues**: Heavy metals like **lead and mercury** impair cognitive function, increasing the risk of Alzheimer's and neurodegenerative diseases.

**Action Step:** Check the ingredients in your personal care products today and remove anything with **parabens, sulfates,** or **artificial fragrances**.

## Steps for Detoxing Your Home, Water, Diet, and Body

The good news? You can *significantly* reduce your toxic load with a few simple changes. Here are some steps to help you begin detoxifying your life:

**Clean Up Your Diet:**

- **Choose organic produce** to minimize pesticide exposure.
- **Avoid processed foods** that contain artificial additives and preservatives.
- **Drink filtered water** to eliminate heavy metals and contaminants.
- **Swap plastic containers for glass** to reduce BPA exposure.

**Detox Your Home:**

- **Replace chemical-laden cleaning products** with natural alternatives like vinegar, baking soda, and essential oils.
- **Use HEPA air filters** to remove airborne toxins.
- **Switch to non-toxic personal care products** – check labels for parabens, sulfates, and synthetic fragrances.

**Detox Your Water:**

Many of the world's water systems rely on 100+-year-old infrastructures, failing to remove modern contaminants. The EPA has identified **over 100 toxins** in public water supplies. Some other common water contaminants include:

- **Lead & Iron**: Leached from aging pipes, contributing to neurological and cardiovascular issues.

- **Chlorine**: Added to disinfect water but can disrupt gut health and oxidative balance.

- **Herbicides & Pesticides**: Agricultural runoff introduces toxic chemicals into water supplies.

- **Fluoride**: Controversial for potential thyroid suppression and metabolic disruption.

**Action Step:** Invest in a high-quality water filter to remove contaminants and ensure clean drinking water.

## Support Your Body's Natural Detox Pathways

Your liver, kidneys, gut, and skin are constantly working to detoxify your body, but they need support to function at their best and avoid being overwhelmed and shutting down. Here's how *you* can enhance your body's natural detoxification process:

- **Hydrate with Lemon Water**: This helps to flush toxins and support kidney function.
- **Eat Cruciferous Vegetables**: Broccoli, kale, and Brussels sprouts help to boost liver detox pathways.
- **Sweat it Out**: Exercise and sauna therapy help to eliminate toxins through the skin.
- **Prioritize Gut Health**: A balanced gut microbiome neutralizes harmful substances.

**Action Step:** Start your day with a glass of warm lemon water to aid detoxification.

# Your 30-Day Action Plan: Detox Reset

Your body is not broken, it's burdened. When you begin to free it from toxins you start to rediscover the vibrant health that was hiding just below the surface. Because toxins are seemingly everywhere they might feel unable to escape, but healing and detoxing is possible. Here's a step-by-step, week-by-week plan to help you begin shedding toxins from your life for the first month:

## WEEK 1: Remove Toxins from Food & Water

- **Swap processed foods** for whole, organic options.
- **Drink filtered** or **spring** water only.

## WEEK 2: Detox Your Home & Personal Care

- **Replace chemical cleaners** with non-toxic alternatives.
- Switch to **paraben- and sulfate-free** personal care products.

## WEEK 3: Support Your Body's Detox Pathways

- Eat **cruciferous vegetables** daily.
- **Incorporate daily movement** to promote circulation.

**WEEK 4: Strengthen Gut Health & Reduce Toxin Exposure**

- **Add probiotic-rich foods** to your diet (fermented foods, yogurt).

- Continue eliminating **plastics & chemical exposure.**

**Action Step:** Pick **one detox habit** and start today!

Your environment plays a *critical* role in your long-term health. By reducing toxic exposure, you empower your body to heal, restore balance, and thrive. I have seen firsthand how reducing toxic exposure can *reverse* chronic disease, restore energy, and help people feel truly *alive* again. The power to heal is already within you. You just need to remove the obstacles in your way.

## Next Up

In **Chapter 8**, we'll explore the science of brain health and how to protect your cognitive function for life.

# Chapter 8:

## Saving Your Brain: Preventing Cognitive Decline Before It's Too Late

## Did You Know? Your Brain Starts Declining Decades Before Symptoms Appear

**Every 3 seconds, someone in the world develops dementia. Alzheimer's is now the fastest-growing epidemic, and nearly two-thirds of those diagnosed are women. But here's the shocking truth: up to 40% of dementia cases are preventable with the right lifestyle changes** (*The Lancet Commission on Dementia Prevention, 2020*).

What if I told you that the symptoms of Alzheimer's and cognitive decline don't begin in your 70s? They can start *decades* earlier, as early as your 30s and 40s. The brain isn't failing on its own: it's *reacting* to years of poor diet, lack of movement, toxic exposure, and chronic stress.

Now, imagine a woman named Emily. At 52, she began forgetting words in conversations and misplacing items. Her doctor brushed it off as "just aging." But Emily *knew* something wasn't right. Instead of accepting this as her fate, she took action: eliminating processed foods, walking daily, and focusing on brain-boosting nutrients. A year later, her memory had improved, her brain fog lifted, and her energy was restored. Cognitive decline is **not** inevitable. You have the power to take control of your brain. Starting today.

Think of your brain as a garden. If you don't nurture it, weeds (inflammation, toxins, poor nutrition) will take over, choking out the healthy plants (your neurons and brain pathways). Conventional medicine only trims the weeds (prescribing drugs), but true healing comes from restoring the soil (proper nutrition, detoxification, and movement).

Neurodegenerative diseases like Alzheimer's have become part of a healthcare model that often emphasizes long-term symptom management over prevention. Medications developed for Alzheimer's may slow the progression of symptoms, but they do not offer a cure; yet they generate billions in revenue.

In contrast, research shows that simple lifestyle shifts, like movement, nutrition, sleep, and mental engagement, could reduce the risk of cognitive decline by up to 40%. Still, these strategies are often underemphasized because they aren't tied to profit in the same way.

This is why it's more important than ever to be informed. You have the power to support your brain health through natural, proactive choices. Starting today.

| Conventional Approach | Root-Cause Approach |
|---|---|
| Treats symptoms with prescription drugs | Prevents cognitive decline through nutrition and lifestyle |
| Focuses on medication to slow disease | Focuses on reducing inflammation and repairing neurons |
| Ignores the role of diet, sleep, and toxins | Addresses gut health, sleep, stress, and movement |
| Recommends outdated dietary advice (low-fat diets) | Promotes brain-supportive foods like healthy fats and antioxidants |

## Myths vs. Truths About Brain Health

| Myth | Truth |
|---|---|
| Dementia is just a part of aging. | Dementia is **not** an inevitable part of aging. Studies show that up to **40% of cases are preventable** with diet, exercise, and lifestyle changes. |
| **Action Step:** Eat brain-boosting foods rich in antioxidants and healthy fats, like wild salmon, blueberries, and walnuts. ||

| Memory loss starts in your 70s. | The brain starts declining decades earlier: your 30s and 40s. Cognitive function depends on how you live today. |
|---|---|
| **Action Step:** Engage in lifelong learning: read, learn new skills, or play an instrument to strengthen neural pathways. ||

| There's nothing you can do once you start experiencing brain fog. | Brain fog is often caused by chronic inflammation and nutrient deficiencies, which are completely reversible with proper nutrition and detoxification. |
|---|---|
| **Action Step:** Cut out sugar and ultra-processed foods for one week and track how your focus and energy improve. ||

## How Inflammation and Metabolic Dysfunction Affect the Brain

Inflammation is often referred to as **the silent killer**, and its effects on the brain are devastating. Chronic inflammation can damage neurons, the brain's essential cells, and disrupt the delicate communication between brain cells. This interference not only accelerates cognitive decline but also contributes to the development of conditions like Alzheimer's and other forms of dementia. Some of the hidden causes of brain inflammation include:

- **High Sugar Intake**: Excess glucose fuels oxidative stress, damaging neurons and increasing the risk of Alzheimer's and dementia.
- **Poor Gut Health**: An unhealthy gut microbiome sends inflammatory signals to the brain, impairing mood, memory, and focus.
- **Insulin Resistance**: Also called "Type 3 Diabetes," poor blood sugar regulation has been linked to cognitive decline.

A *Nature Neuroscience* study found that chronic inflammation in the brain is a key driver of neurodegeneration. The good news? Reducing inflammation through lifestyle changes can significantly protect and restore brain function.

**Action Step:** Cut refined sugar and processed foods from your diet for one week and track how your focus and mental clarity improve.

## The Link Between Alzheimer's, Dementia, and Lifestyle Choices

Alzheimer's and dementia don't happen randomly, they develop over decades due to a combination of lifestyle and environmental factors. A groundbreaking study published in *The Lancet* identified key modifiable risk factors that significantly influence dementia risk, including:

- **Lack of Physical Activity**: Regular movement boosts brain-derived neurotrophic factor (BDNF), a protein essential for neuroplasticity.
- **Sleep Deprivation**: Poor sleep accelerates beta-amyloid plaque buildup, a hallmark of Alzheimer's.
- **Chronic Stress**: Persistent stress shrinks the hippocampus, the brain's memory center.

**Action Step:** Set a consistent sleep schedule: aim for 7 to 9 hours per night to support cognitive recovery.

## Brain-Boosting Foods and Supplements

Your brain requires specific nutrients to function at its best. Eating nutrient-dense foods can enhance cognitive function, protect neurons from damage, and even support the growth of new brain cells. A diet rich in antioxidants, healthy fats, vitamins, and minerals helps reduce inflammation, improve memory, and sharpen focus, playing a crucial role in long-term brain health.

**Best Foods for Brain Health:**

- **Fatty Fish (Salmon, Mackerel)**: Rich in **omega-3 fatty acids** that reduce inflammation and support brain cell membranes.
- **Leafy Greens (Spinach, Kale)**: Packed with **antioxidants and vitamin K**, which protect against cognitive decline.
- **Berries (Blueberries, Blackberries)**: Contain **anthocyanins** that enhance memory and slow brain aging.
- **Nuts & Seeds (Walnuts, Flaxseeds)**: Provide **vitamin E**, a powerful antioxidant that protects brain cells.
- **Turmeric**: Contains **curcumin**, which crosses the blood-brain barrier to **reduce inflammation and support cognitive function**.

**Top Brain-Supporting Supplements:**

- **Omega-3 Fatty Acids**: Essential for **reducing brain inflammation** and improving mental clarity.
- **Magnesium**: Supports **neurotransmitter function** and helps regulate stress response.
- **Lion's Mane Mushroom**: Shown to **stimulate nerve growth factor (NGF)** and promote brain cell regeneration.

- **B Vitamins**: Critical for **energy production and reducing homocysteine levels** linked to brain atrophy.

**Action Step:** Add **one brain-boosting food** to your diet today.

*Any nutritional or supplement recommendations are intended to support general wellness and are not meant to diagnose, treat, or prevent any disease. Consult your healthcare provider before starting any diet or supplement program.

## Daily Habits to Improve Memory, Focus, and Prevent Cognitive Decline

Optimizing brain health goes beyond diet: it's about adopting daily habits that actively support and strengthen cognitive function. Simple lifestyle changes, such as regular exercise, quality sleep, stress management, and lifelong learning, can enhance mental clarity, boost memory, and promote long-term brain resilience. By making these habits part of your routine, you can significantly improve both mental clarity and overall longevity.

**Prioritize Deep Sleep:**
- Sleep is when the brain **detoxifies and consolidates memories**. Aim for **7 to 9 hours per night** to optimize cognitive recovery.

**Engage in Lifelong Learning:**

- Activities like **reading, learning a new language, or playing an instrument** strengthen neural pathways and enhance cognitive resilience.

**Move Your Body:**

- Physical exercise is one of the **most effective ways to protect brain health**. Aerobic workouts **increase blood flow**, while strength training promotes **neuroprotective compounds**.

**Manage Stress Effectively:**

- Chronic stress **damages brain cells** and impairs memory. Practice **mindfulness, deep breathing, or meditation** to lower cortisol levels.

**Foster Social Connections:**

- Strong social ties **lower the risk of dementia**. Engage in meaningful conversations, join community groups, and **prioritize relationships**.

**Action Step:** Spend **at least 10 minutes today** on an activity that challenges your brain (reading, learning, or solving puzzles).

# How to Reverse Cognitive Decline and Boost Brain Health

## 1. Reduce Brain Inflammation with an Anti-Inflammatory Diet:

**Eat more:**
- Omega-3-rich foods (wild salmon, flaxseeds, walnuts)
- Leafy greens and cruciferous vegetables (broccoli, spinach)
- Berries (blueberries, blackberries)
- Turmeric and ginger (anti-inflammatory spices)

**Avoid:**
- Processed foods, refined sugars, and industrial seed oils
- Artificial sweeteners, which disrupt gut-brain communication
- Excess alcohol and ultra-processed snacks

**Action Step:** Add **one brain-boosting food** to your meals today.

## 2. Optimize Sleep to Detox Your Brain

Did you know your brain flushes out toxins **while you sleep**? This is why poor sleep **increases your risk of Alzheimer's**.

**How to Improve Sleep for Brain Health:**

- Stick to a consistent bedtime and wake-up schedule.
- Reduce blue light exposure before bed.
- Take magnesium and melatonin for deeper sleep.

**Action Step:** Set an alarm **30 minutes before bed** to start winding down.

### 3. Move Daily for Brain Function

Exercise **increases blood flow** to the brain, boosts **brain-derived neurotrophic factor (BDNF)** and reduces cognitive decline.

**Best Types of Movement for Brain Health:**

- **Strength Training** – Builds muscle, balances hormones, and improves brain function.
- **Aerobic Exercise** – Increases oxygen supply to the brain.
- **Yoga & Tai Chi** – Reduces stress and inflammation.

**Action Step:** Walk for **10 minutes after meals** to increase blood flow to the brain.

## 4. Manage Stress to Protect Your Memory

How to Lower Stress Naturally:

- **Deep breathing exercises** (4-7-8 technique)
- **Daily gratitude practice** to shift your mindset
- **Adaptogenic herbs** like Ashwagandha and Rhodiola

**Action Step:** Spend **5 minutes in meditation or deep breathing today.**

# Your 30-Day Action Plan: Brain Optimization

By incorporating brain-boosting foods, engaging in regular exercise, prioritizing quality rest, and reducing inflammation, you can start supporting your overall cognitive resilience. This week-by-week, step-by-step approach will empower you with easy, accessible steps to start taking control of your brain health to create lasting, positive change starting today:

### WEEK 1: Nutrition & Hydration

- Add **brain-boosting foods** (fatty fish, leafy greens, berries) to your diet.

- Drink **filtered water** to eliminate contaminants affecting brain function.

### WEEK 2: Sleep & Stress Management

- Set a **consistent bedtime** and wake-up schedule.

- Practice **deep breathing or meditation** daily.

### WEEK 3: Movement & Learning

- Engage in **at least 30 minutes of exercise daily**.

- Read, learn a new skill, or engage in a mentally stimulating activity.

## WEEK 4: Strengthening Cognitive Resilience

- Prioritize **social connections** and meaningful conversations.

- Continue daily brain-boosting habits for **long-term health**.

**Action Step:** Choose **one habit to start today** and track your progress over the next 30 days!

Your brain health is in your hands. I have seen how by eating the right foods, staying active, managing stress, and prioritizing mental stimulation, you can sharpen your memory, improve focus, and reduce the risk of neurodegenerative diseases. This is *your* moment, start taking action now. Your brain deserves it.

## Next Up

In **Chapter 9**, we'll explore the link between obesity and metabolic dysfunction: how to break the cycle of weight gain and disease.

Chapter 9:

# Conquering Obesity: End the Struggle for Good

## Did You Know? Obesity is More Than Just Willpower

**Obesity now surpasses smoking as the leading cause of preventable death, contributing to heart disease, diabetes, and cancer. Nearly 75% of U.S. adults are overweight or obese, yet 95% of diets fail in the long run. Why? Because obesity is not just a calorie problem: it's a metabolic disease** (*Journal of the American Medical Association, 2021*).

For years, people like David were told that weight loss was simply about "eating less and moving more." At 47, he had tried every diet, from low-fat to keto, only to regain the weight each time. Frustrated and exhausted, he searched for real answers. That's when he discovered the root cause of his struggle: **insulin resistance** was keeping his body in fat-storage mode, his **gut bacteria** were out of balance, and **chronic stress** was sabotaging his metabolism. Instead of following another restrictive diet, David focused on hormonal healing, metabolic flexibility, and gut restoration. Within a year, he lost 60 pounds, reversed his prediabetes, and finally felt in control of his health. The key to lasting weight loss *isn't* starvation. It's metabolic restoration.

Imagine your body as a home with a thermostat that regulates temperature. When functioning properly, it adjusts heating and cooling to keep the home comfortable. But when it malfunctions, the house may become too hot (fat storage) or too cold (a sluggish metabolism). Obesity *isn't* about willpower; it's about repairing this broken internal thermostat, which is controlled by insulin, hormones, and metabolism. Once restored, your body can naturally maintain a healthy weight without the need for extreme dieting or deprivation.

Obesity-related conditions represent a $200 billion market, and much of the current system focuses on managing symptoms rather than addressing root causes like metabolic dysfunction, diet, and lifestyle.

Weight-loss medications are often prescribed without tackling the underlying imbalances that drive weight gain.

Bariatric surgery has become increasingly common, yet long-term success still depends on sustainable lifestyle changes. And while medications like Ozempic and Metformin generate billions annually, evidence shows that type 2 diabetes can often be reversed through targeted lifestyle interventions.

This is why informed, proactive choices matter. When individuals understand their options and take a whole-person approach, they can begin to break the cycle, and reclaim their health.

| Conventional Approach | Root-Cause Approach |
|---|---|
| Focuses on calorie restriction | Focuses on hormone balance and metabolism |
| Recommends low-fat, high-carb diets | Prioritizes whole foods and nutrient-dense fats |
| Treats symptoms with weight-loss drugs | Reverses insulin resistance for natural fat loss |
| Blames willpower | Fixes metabolic dysfunction |

## Myths vs. Truths About Obesity

| Myth | Truth |
|---|---|
| Weight gain is just about eating too many calories. | Obesity is a hormonal disorder, not just a calorie problem. Insulin, leptin, and cortisol determine fat storage more than calorie intake. |
| **Action Step:** Reduce processed carbs and sugar for one week to improve insulin function. ||

| Obesity is caused by lack of willpower. | Leptin resistance tricks the brain into thinking you're starving. When leptin is out of balance, you constantly feel hungry, no matter how much you eat. |
|---|---|
| **Action Step:** Eat more protein and fiber to regulate leptin and reduce cravings. ||

| Exercise is the key to weight loss. | Exercise supports weight loss, but fixing metabolism is what makes it sustainable. 80% of weight loss is determined by diet, sleep, and hormones, not just workouts. |
|---|---|
| **Action Step:** Focus on strength training (2 to 3 times per week) to improve insulin sensitivity. ||

## Hormones, Metabolism & Gut Health: The Hidden Drivers of Weight Gain

Hormones, metabolism, and gut health all play a crucial role in weight regulation, often more than calories alone. Imbalances in insulin, cortisol can lead to fat storage and slow metabolism, while an unhealthy gut can trigger inflammation and cravings. A *Diabetes Care* study found that insulin resistance appears before weight gain, proving that metabolic dysfunction is a root cause of obesity, not just a side effect.

**Key Factors That Influence Fat Storage:**

- **Insulin Resistance**: High insulin levels **lock fat in storage mode**, making weight loss impossible.

- **Leptin Resistance**: Leptin signals fullness, but when disrupted, the brain **thinks you're starving**, leading to cravings.

- **Chronic Stress & Cortisol**: Cortisol raises blood sugar and **stores fat around the belly**.

- **Gut Microbiome Imbalance**: An unhealthy gut **increases fat absorption and inflammation**.

## Why Conventional Diets Fail: The Truth About Metabolism

Most people believe weight loss is simply a matter of willpower, but the *real* reason diets fail is that they slow down metabolism. Better understanding your metabolism, and the factors that effect it, will help you achieve sustainable weight loss.

**The Science of Metabolic Slowdown:**

- Extreme calorie restriction **slows your metabolic rate** (New England Journal of Medicine, 2016).

- Cutting too many carbs without a strategy leads to **hormonal imbalances** and **muscle loss**.

- Rebound weight gain happens when leptin levels drop, **making you hungrier** and **storing more fat**.

**Solution:** Instead of dieting, focus on metabolic healing: balancing insulin, reducing inflammation, and restoring gut health.

## Get a Second Opinion

While on your journey to sustainable weight loss, consider partnering with **weight loss clinics, nutritionists, or functional medicine providers** who offer natural, personalized solutions rather than relying solely on medications or invasive procedures.

Unlike conventional approaches, these specialists focus on addressing the underlying hormonal, metabolic, and gut health issues that cause weight gain. By working with professionals who utilize nutritional guidance, lifestyle coaching, and targeted supplementation, you can safely achieve your weight loss goals while optimizing overall health.

Embracing these holistic methods empowers you with sustainable habits, reduces risk of relapsing into unhealthy habits or behaviors, and sets the stage for lifelong wellness.

## The Missing Nutrients: How Amino Acids & L-Carnitine Unlock Fat Loss

Our modern food system has stripped away essential amino acids needed for fat metabolism.

**Essential amino acids** are amino acids that your body cannot produce on its own and must therefore be obtained through the foods you eat or dietary supplements. They play critical roles in building proteins, maintaining muscle mass, supporting hormone production, and regulating metabolic processes.

There are nine essential amino acids: **histidine, isoleucine, leucine, lysine, methionine, phenylalanine, threonine, tryptophan, and valine.**

Without adequate intake of these amino acids, the body struggles to perform vital functions, potentially leading to muscle loss, weakened immunity, and impaired overall health.

Among the **essential amino acids**, several can play key roles in combating obesity and promoting weight management. Specifically, these essential amino acids are especially beneficial:

## Three Essential Amino Acids to Reduce Obesity

1. Leucine:

- **Role:** Helps regulate metabolism, maintain muscle mass, and promote fat loss.

- **How it combats obesity:** Leucine stimulates protein synthesis and preserves lean muscle tissue during weight loss, thereby enhancing your metabolic rate and improving fat burning.

2. Isoleucine:

- **Role:** Supports energy regulation and fat metabolism.

- **How it combats obesity:** Helps maintain stable blood sugar levels, reducing hunger and cravings, and supports better utilization of stored fats as energy.

3. Valine

- **Role:** Important for muscle metabolism and energy production.

- **How it combats obesity:** Aids in maintaining muscle mass during calorie restriction, preventing metabolic slowdown associated with dieting.

Together, these three (**leucine**, **isoleucine**, and **valine**) are known as **Branched-Chain Amino Acids (BCAAs)**, which are particularly beneficial for enhancing metabolism, maintaining muscle during weight loss, and facilitating fat burning.

Incorporate a high-quality source of BCAAs into your diet, either through natural sources (like eggs, lean meats, fish, legumes), or supplementation to enhance weight-loss efforts and metabolism naturally.

**How L-Carnitine Helps Burn Fat:**

- **Breaks down stored fat** and shrinks fat cells.
- **Activates brown fat**, which generates heat and increases calorie                                                        burning.
  **Boosts energy** by enhancing mitochondrial function which boosts metabolism and fat burning.

**How to Restore Fat-Burning Nutrients:**

- **Eat L-Carnitine-rich foods** (grass-fed meat, wild fish, dairy).
- **Supplement with amino acids** to restore nutrient balance. **Incorporate thermogenic foods** (green tea, chili peppers, coconut oil) to accelerate metabolism.

# The Science of Sustainable Fat Loss: What Actually Works

By now we understand that it's not "quick-fixes" or "miracle drugs" that help us lose & keep weight off, it's sustainable practices and overall lifestyle changes. By focusing on long-term habits rather than short-term restrictions, you can achieve lasting weight loss and overall health.

A few scientifically proven sustainable fat loss methods include:

### 1. Fix Insulin Resistance:

- **Reduce processed carbs & sugar** to stabilize blood sugar.
- **Try intermittent fasting** (12 to 16 hour fasting windows) to improve insulin function.
- **Prioritize strength training** to enhance insulin sensitivity.

## 2. Balance Gut Health for Weight Control:

- **Eat probiotic-rich foods** (yogurt, kimchi, sauerkraut) for a healthier gut microbiome.
- **Increase fiber intake** (chia seeds, flaxseeds, leafy greens) to nourish good bacteria.
- **Avoid artificial sweeteners**, which disrupt gut bacteria and cause cravings.

## 3. Manage Stress & Sleep to Prevent Fat Storage:

- **Practice stress reduction** (meditation, deep breathing, nature walks).
- **Prioritize 7 to 9 hours of quality sleep**, poor sleep raises cortisol and promotes weight gain.

## 4. Move in a Way That Supports Metabolism:

- **Strength train 2 to 3 times a week** to build muscle and increase resting metabolism.
- **Walk after meals** to regulate blood sugar.
- **Incorporate HIIT workouts** for maximum fat burn.

# Fasting: A Powerful Tool to End Obesity

Fasting has emerged as a powerful tool in the fight against obesity, helping to reset metabolism, enhance fat burning, and regulate insulin levels. By giving your body strategic breaks from eating, **fasting encourages it to use stored fat as fuel, promoting sustainable weight loss and improved metabolic health**.

While fasting might seem daunting initially, its benefits extend beyond weight loss, also enhancing cellular repair and longevity. Later in this book, we'll dive deeper into fasting methods, their specific benefits, and how to safely integrate fasting into your daily routine to effectively combat obesity and regain control of your health.

# Your 30-Day Action Plan: Metabolic Reset

Weight loss is a complex and often sensitive topic in our society. Many people hope for quick fixes, but true, healthy weight loss takes time, commitment, and the right strategy. The good news? It doesn't have to be expensive, risky, or overwhelming. This step-by-step, week-by-week approach will provide simple, effective strategies to help you regain control of your metabolism and achieve sustainable, healthy weight loss:

## WEEK 1: Improve Insulin Sensitivity

- Cut out refined sugars and processed foods.
- Start a 12-hour fasting window (ex: 8 PM - 8 AM).

## WEEK 2: Heal the Gut Microbiome

- Eat probiotic and prebiotic-rich foods daily.
- Increase fiber intake to support digestion.

## WEEK 3: Optimize Fat-Burning Hormones

- Incorporate strength training and walking after meals.
- Practice stress management techniques.

## WEEK 4: Sustain & Maintain Your Progress

- Continue eating nutrient-dense, whole foods.

- Prioritize deep sleep and daily movement.

**Action Step:** Choose **one habit** from the reset plan and start today!

Obesity is *not* just about willpower: it's about balancing hormones, fixing metabolism, and restoring nutrient deficiencies. I have seen firsthand that when you reset your body's internal weight-regulation system, fat loss happens naturally and sustainably. Your health is your birthright; you don't have to wait for permission to take it back.

**Next Up**

In **Chapter 10**, we'll uncover how to heal chronic pain without relying on medication in order to reclaim a pain-free life.

# Chapter 10:

## Pain Relief Without Pills: Healing Chronic Pain and Inflammation Naturally

Did You Know? Chronic Pain is the #1 Cause of Disability Worldwide

**More than 50 million Americans suffer from chronic pain, making it the leading cause of disability globally. Shockingly, over 80% of these cases could be managed or reversed with lifestyle interventions, yet painkillers remain the primary treatment** (*Journal of Pain Research, 2022*)**.**

For years, Rachel suffered from debilitating back pain. Doctors prescribed opioids, recommended physical therapy, and even considered surgery, but nothing provided lasting relief. As her dependence on medication grew, so did her pain. Frustrated and searching for answers, Rachel turned to a functional medicine approach. She discovered that her pain was driven by chronic inflammation, poor posture, and unaddressed emotional stress. Through chiropractic care, an anti-inflammatory diet, nutritional supplements and daily movement, she *fully* healed, *without* medication. Chronic pain isn't something you *have* to accept. You can heal, and I'll show you how.

**Pain is your body's built-in alarm system,** signaling that something is wrong. But what happens when the alarm never shuts off? Imagine a fire alarm blaring nonstop, even when there's no fire. Painkillers may muffle the noise, but they don't address the underlying problem. True healing requires identifying and eliminating the source of the pain, not just silencing the symptoms. To put out the fire, and finally disable the alarm, you must first find what's fueling it.

**Chronic pain costs the U.S. economy over $635 billion annually**, and much of the current system focuses on managing pain rather than resolving its root causes.

Pain medications, including opioids and NSAIDs, can offer short-term relief but often don't address underlying issues like inflammation or structural imbalances.

Surgical procedures such as spinal fusions are common, yet many patients continue to struggle if muscle imbalances, metabolic dysfunction, or inflammation aren't addressed.

This is why taking a whole-person, integrative approach, alongside conventional care, can be a powerful way forward. When you become informed, you can explore safe, supportive options that go beyond masking symptoms and move toward real healing.

| Conventional Approach | Root-Cause Approach |
|---|---|
| Use painkillers to mask symptoms | Addresses the underlying cause of pain |
| Focuses on symptom suppression | Focuses on reducing inflammation naturally |
| Recommends surgery for chronic conditions | Uses physical therapy, chiropractic, and lifestyle healing |
| Relies on opioids and NSAIDs | Uses nutrition, movement, and holistic therapies |

**The truth?** Chronic pain is a business, and the system isn't designed to heal you. But you can take control.

# Myths vs. Truths About Chronic Pain

| Myth | Truth |
|---|---|
| If you're in pain, you should rest and avoid movement. | Too much rest worsens pain. Movement reduces stiffness, improves circulation, and strengthens muscles. |
| **Action Step:** Try gentle stretching or walking today to reduce stiffness and promote healing. ||

| Painkillers are the only way to manage chronic pain. | Painkillers don't heal pain, they numb it. Long-term use can actually increase pain sensitivity. |
|---|---|
| **Action Step:** Reduce reliance on NSAIDs or opioids by incorporating natural anti-inflammatory foods like turmeric and omega-3s. ||

| Chronic pain is a normal part of aging. | Pain is not an inevitable part of getting older. Many people reverse chronic pain by addressing posture, nutrition, inflammation, and movement. |
|---|---|
| **Action Step:** Focus on daily mobility exercises to maintain flexibility and reduce joint stiffness. ||

# The Real Causes of Chronic Pain

Chronic pain isn't just the result of a past injury: it's often fueled by ongoing inflammation, nerve dysfunction, and muscle imbalances. Identifying the underlying cause, whether it's systemic inflammation, compressed nerves, or postural strain, is the first and most crucial step toward lasting relief and healing.

**Key Contributors to Chronic Pain:**

**Chronic Inflammation**: Long-term inflammation sensitizes nerves, making pain worse. Studies in *The Journal of Clinical Investigation* link inflammation to conditions like arthritis, fibromyalgia, and autoimmune disorders.

**Nerve Dysfunction**: Damaged or overstimulated nerves can cause pain to persist, even after an injury heals. Conditions such as neuropathy are often driven by poor metabolic health and inflammation.

**Musculoskeletal Imbalances**: Poor posture, weak core muscles, and prolonged sitting strain the body, leading to chronic back, neck, and joint pain.

# Why Painkillers Aren't the Answer (And Can Make Things Worse)

While painkillers can provide temporary relief, they do not resolve the underlying causes of pain. Instead, they mask symptoms, allowing the real issues to persist and worsen. Over time, reliance on medication can have severe consequences.

**The Hidden Risks of Painkillers:**

- **Masking the Problem**: Instead of fixing the underlying dysfunction, painkillers dull the pain, allowing conditions to worsen over time.

- **Increased Sensitivity to Pain**: *The Journal of Neuroscience* found that long-term opioid use actually increases pain sensitivity, creating a cycle of dependency.

- **Serious Side Effects**: NSAIDs can cause stomach ulcers, liver damage, and heart complications, while opioids carry risks of addiction and cognitive impairment.

**Action Step:** If you rely on daily painkillers, start exploring natural pain management strategies to reduce dependency.

## Healing Chronic Pain by Addressing Inflammation

Instead of merely **masking pain**, a holistic approach to healing **reduces inflammation** at the source. Key strategies to heal chronic pain by addressing inflammation include:

**Eliminating Common Inflammatory Triggers:**
- Processed foods, refined sugar, and trans fats
- Chronic stress and poor sleep
- Environmental toxins and lack of movement

**Incorporating an Anti-Inflammatory Solution:**
- **Eat Whole, Nutrient-Dense Foods**: Omega-3-rich foods (wild-caught fish, flaxseeds), turmeric, and leafy greens.
- **Move Your Body Daily**: Walking, yoga, and strength training improve circulation and relieve stiffness.
- **Manage Stress Effectively**: Meditation, breathwork, and acupuncture lower cortisol and inflammation levels.

## The Role of Chiropractic Care, Physical Therapy & Natural Health Sciences

Chiropractic care, physical therapy, and alternative healing methods play a crucial role in addressing the root causes of pain and restoring body function. Together, these therapies offer a holistic path to lasting pain relief and improved well-being.

- **Chiropractic Adjustments**: Realign the spine to reduce nerve irritation and improve mobility. A study in *The Journal of Manipulative and Physiological Therapeutics* found chiropractic care **more effective than medication** for chronic back pain.

- **Physical Therapy & Corrective Exercise**: Strengthen weak muscles, improve posture, and restore movement patterns. Techniques like **myofascial release** are a hands-on therapy technique that applies gentle, sustained pressure to relieve tension, tightness, and pain within the connective tissues (fascia) surrounding muscles. This type of therapy can help retrain the body to move efficiently.

- **Acupuncture**: Stimulate the body's natural pain-relief mechanisms and reduce stress-related pain.

- **Mind-Body Therapies:** Enhance the mind's ability to positively influence physical health and manage symptoms like chronic pain, anxiety, and inflammation. They are practices that focus on the interaction between your mental, emotional, and physical well-being, helping to promote relaxation, reduce stress, and support overall health and healing. Examples include **meditation, guided imagery, deep-breathing exercises, yoga, tai chi, biofeedback,** and **progressive muscle relaxation.**

**Action Step:** Try **one alternative therapy** this month: chiropractic, acupuncture, or physical therapy to see how it impacts your pain levels.

## Cutting-Edge Solutions: How Stem Cells Reduce Chronic Inflammation & Pain

Pain and inflammation are closely linked, with chronic inflammation being a major contributor to long-term pain conditions. When inflammation becomes persistent, it disrupts the body's natural healing processes, leading to ongoing discomfort and tissue damage. Emerging research points to **Mesenchymal Stem Cells (MSCs)** as a groundbreaking approach to naturally managing inflammation and promoting recovery. These specialized cells offer new hope for those struggling with chronic pain.

## How MSC Therapy Works

**Regulates Immune Response**: MSCs communicate with immune cells to calm an overactive inflammatory response, helping to restore balance.

**Suppresses Pro-Inflammatory Cytokines**: MSCs lower key inflammatory markers like TNF-α, IL-6, and IL-1β, which are known to fuel chronic pain and tissue damage.

**Promotes Tissue Regeneration**: These powerful cells release growth factors that aid in repairing muscles, joints, and nerves, supporting long-term healing and pain relief.

**Conditions That Benefit from MSC Therapy:**

- **Arthritis & Joint Pain**
- **Autoimmune Diseases:** Rheumatoid Arthritis, MS, Lupus
- **Neurodegenerative Conditions:** Alzheimer's, Parkinson's

- **Metabolic Disorders:** Diabetes, Obesity-Related Inflammation

*The science in MSC is evolving, and the information presented should not be interpreted as conclusive or as a replacement for professional medical guidance.

# Your 30-Day Action Plan: Chronic Pain Reset

Pain is not something you have to live with; it's not something that you should have to over medicate yourself to deal with. When in the throws of chronic pain, it's hard to imagine a path to recovery, but it *is* possible through natural, holistic lifestyle changes. This step-by-step, week-by-week approach will provide an initial gameplan to help you beat chronic pain:

## WEEK 1: Reduce Inflammatory Triggers

- Swap **processed foods** for whole, nutrient-dense options.
- Begin a **daily stretching and mobility routine**.

## WEEK 2: Incorporate Natural Pain Relievers

- Add **turmeric, ginger, and omega-3-rich foods** to meals.
- Try **chiropractic care, acupuncture, or massage therapy**.

## WEEK 3: Improve Sleep & Stress Management

- Establish a **consistent bedtime routine**.
- Incorporate **breathwork, meditation, or nature walks**.

**WEEK 4: Strengthen & Support Healing**

- Engage in **strength training or yoga** to support posture.
- Reduce **screen time and avoid prolonged sitting**.

I have seen that by addressing inflammation, movement, posture, and mindset, you *can* break free from chronic pain and inflammation without medication. Breaking out of this constant pain cycle is possible, you do not have to live with a persistent pain alarm ringing in your brain.

## Next Up

In **Chapter 11**, we'll explore how to reverse and prevent diabetes through diet, exercise, and metabolic healing.

# Chapter 11:

## Beat Diabetes: A Proven Plan

## Did You Know? Diabetes Was Once Rare. Now It's an Epidemic

**More than 537 million adults worldwide have diabetes, and by 2045, that number is projected to reach 783 million. Even more shocking? Nearly 1 in 3 adults has prediabetes and doesn't even know it** (*International Diabetes Federation, 2023*).

For years, Carlos struggled with Type 2 diabetes, believing it was a lifelong condition. His doctors told him he would need daily medication indefinitely, and he resigned himself to worsening health. But everything changed when he took control of his diet, incorporated fasting, and made movement a priority. In just six months, he *reversed* his diabetes symptoms: no more medication, no more blood sugar spikes.

Carlos isn't an exception; he's *proof* that with the right lifestyle changes, Type 2 diabetes can put into remission. Imagine a bustling highway designed to keep traffic moving efficiently. Insulin acts as the traffic cop, directing cars (glucose) into parking spots (cells) where they can be used for energy. But when insulin resistance develops, it's like the traffic signals are broken: cars pile up, causing gridlock, just as excess sugar accumulates in the bloodstream.

Instead of repairing the traffic system (insulin sensitivity), conventional treatments often just add more lanes (medications like insulin or Metformin) without addressing the root issue. The real solution? Fixing the signals. By improving insulin sensitivity through diet, movement, and lifestyle changes, you can restore proper metabolic function. You don't need *more* lanes: you need to clear the roadblocks and let your body's natural system work as it was designed to.

A hundred years ago, Type 2 diabetes was rare. Today, nearly 1 in 10 adults has it, and the numbers continue to rise. So, what changed? It's not our genetics; our DNA hasn't shifted that quickly. The real culprits are our modern environment, highly processed diets, and sedentary lifestyles.

**However, diabetes doesn't have to be a life sentence.** Unlike Type 1 diabetes, which is an autoimmune disorder, Type 2 diabetes is largely caused by lifestyle factors: meaning it may be both preventable and reversible. Yet, conventional treatments focus on managing blood sugar rather than fixing the root cause: **insulin resistance.**

**Diabetes-related healthcare costs exceed \$760 billion annually**: largely due to a system focused on managing symptoms rather than reversing the condition. Rather than addressing root causes like insulin resistance through lifestyle change, treatment often centers on long-term medication.

Meanwhile, popular nutrition messaging, such as low-fat, high-carb diets, can unintentionally worsen blood sugar imbalances. Medications like Metformin and insulin play a role in care, but they don't solve the underlying metabolic dysfunction for many patients.

That's why being informed is so important. Research shows that type 2 diabetes can often be prevented, or even reversed, through integrative lifestyle strategies. When individuals take an active role in their health, better outcomes become possible.

| Conventional Approach | Root-Cause Approach |
|---|---|
| Prescribes lifelong medication | Focuses on reversing insulin resistance |

| | |
|---|---|
| Promotes high-carb, low-fat diets | Recommends whole foods and low-carb nutrition |
| Treats symptoms (high blood sugar) | Fixes the cause (insulin resistance) |
| Encourages calorie restriction | Supports metabolic healing through fasting and strength training |

## Myths vs. Truths About Diabetes

| Myth | Truth |
|---|---|
| Diabetes is genetic: there's nothing you can do about it. | Only about 10% of diabetes cases are genetic. The other 90% are lifestyle-driven (*Harvard School of Public Health*). |
| **Action Step:** Shift your focus from "genetics" to daily habits: nutrition, movement, and stress reduction can transform your health. | |

| | |
|---|---|
| You just need to eat fewer calories to control diabetes. | Calorie restriction doesn't fix insulin resistance. It's more about food quality than quantity. |
| **Action Step:** Swap refined carbs for whole, fiber-rich foods to improve blood sugar stability. | |

| If you have diabetes, you must take medication for life. | Thousands of people have reversed diabetes naturally. Medication is a short-term tool, not a lifelong requirement. |
|---|---|

**Action Step:** Work with a healthcare provider to create a medication-reduction plan through diet and lifestyle changes.

## The Hidden Cause of Diabetes: Insulin Resistance

Think of insulin as a key that unlocks your cells, allowing glucose to enter and be used for energy. However, when we consume too much sugar, refined carbs, and processed foods, our cells become less responsive to insulin. This is insulin resistance: the real, underlying cause of Type 2 diabetes. Type 2 diabetes can sneak up on you, but there are several warning signs to look out for, including:

- Constant sugar cravings
- Fatigue after eating
- Belly fat that won't go away
- Brain fog
- High blood pressure
- Skin tags or dark patches on the skin

A study in *The Lancet* found that **90% of Type 2 diabetes cases** could be prevented or reversed through lifestyle changes alone.

Yet, conventional medicine focuses on treating the symptom (high blood sugar) instead of fixing the cause (insulin resistance).

## Why Conventional Diabetes Treatments Are Failing Us

Most doctors prescribe lifelong medication to treat diabetes without addressing the root cause of why the insulin resistance is happening to begin with. Here's why this approach is flawed:

- **Medications don't fix insulin resistance.** They simply lower blood sugar without restoring proper glucose metabolism.

- **Standard diabetes diets are outdated.** The American Diabetes Association recommends high-carb diets that spike blood                                                      sugar.

- **Patients become dependent on medication.** Drugs like Metformin and insulin injections mask the problem instead of reversing it.

**The truth?** A *Journal of Clinical Nutrition* study found that low-carb, high-healthy-fat diets were significantly more effective at reversing diabetes than conventional approaches.

# How to Reverse Diabetes Naturally – A Science-Backed Approach

Rather than managing diabetes, let's *reverse* it. With consistent effort, these lifestyle changes can not only stabilize your blood sugar but also eliminate the need for medication, reversing Type 2 diabetes over time. These four strategies have been proven to restore insulin sensitivity and eliminate Type 2 diabetes:

## 1. Adopt a Low-Carb, High-Healthy-Fat Diet:

- **What to Eat:** Healthy fats (avocados, nuts, olive oil), fiber-rich vegetables, grass-fed meats, and wild-caught fish.
- **What to Avoid:** Refined grains, added sugars, industrial seed oils.
  **Science Fact:** A study in *Diabetes Care* found that a low-carb diet improved insulin sensitivity by 75% in just six weeks!

## 2. Prioritize Strength Training & Daily Movement:

- **Strength training** builds muscle, which improves glucose metabolism.
- **Walking after meals** lowers blood sugar and improves insulin response.

- **HIIT workouts** increase insulin sensitivity faster than steady-state cardio.
  **Science Fact:** Just 20 minutes of resistance training three times a week reduces diabetes risk by nearly 50% (*Harvard School of Public Health*).

## 3. Heal the Gut – The Hidden Key to Blood Sugar Balance:

- **Eat more:** Fermented foods (kimchi, sauerkraut, yogurt), prebiotic fiber (garlic, onions, asparagus).
- **Avoid:** Artificial sweeteners, which disrupt gut bacteria and worsen insulin resistance.

  **Science Fact:** People with diabetes have different gut bacteria than those without, proving the gut's role in blood sugar regulation (*Nature Medicine*).

## 4. Improve Sleep & Reduce Stress to Lower Cortisol:

- **Lack of sleep spikes blood sugar.** Aim for 7 to 9 hours of quality rest.
- **Chronic stress raises cortisol, worsening insulin resistance.** Meditation, deep breathing, and nature walks lower cortisol naturally.

**Science Fact:** A *JAMA* *Internal* *Medicine* study found that people who sleep less than 6 hours per night have a 48% higher risk of developing diabetes.

# Your 30-Day Action Plan: Diabetes Reset

If you're struggling with Type 2 diabetes, or even prediabetes, understand that it's not a diagnosis that you can't reverse with diet and lifestyle changes. This step-by-step, week-by-week approach will help you to start fighting back against Type 2 diabetes:

## WEEK 1: Cut Processed Carbs & Sugar

- Swap refined grains for whole foods.

## WEEK 2: Walk After Meals & Strength Train

- Just 10 to 20 minutes makes a difference.

## WEEK 3: Improve Sleep & Manage Stress

- Prioritize deep rest and relaxation.

## WEEK 4: Optimize Gut Health

- Eat fiber, fermented foods, and prebiotics daily.

**Action Step:** Start **one new habit today** to take control of your blood sugar. Small changes lead to big results.

Type 2 diabetes isn't a life sentence: it's a lifestyle condition that may be reversed or prevented. I have seen that by shifting from symptom management to root cause healing, you can take back control of your health, energy, and longevity.

**Next Up**

In **Chapter 12**, we'll explore cutting-edge anti-aging strategies that promote longevity, vitality, and disease-free living.

# Chapter 12:

## Age in Reverse: Secrets for Longevity and Vitality

Did You Know? Aging Is Not Just About Time. It's About Cellular Health

**The average person spends the last 10 years of their life in poor health, battling chronic disease, pain, and declining mobility. But research shows that 80% of this decline is preventable.**

We've been conditioned to believe that aging automatically means frailty, memory loss, and disease. But science now reveals that aging is largely driven by lifestyle, not just genetics: meaning we have far more control over how we age than we once thought.

At 70, Richard felt trapped in his own body. After his doctor prescribed yet another medication, this time for high blood pressure, he struggled with joint pain, low energy, and brain fog. Believing his best years were behind him, he had resigned himself to the inevitable decline of aging. But everything changed when his grandson asked, "Grandpa, will you race me to the tree?" Richard couldn't keep up, and that moment hit him harder than *any* diagnosis. Determined to take control of his health, Richard overhauled his habits, prioritizing nutrition, strength training, fasting, and cold therapy. Within a year, his joint pain vanished, his energy returned, and he stopped taking medication. He even raced his grandson to the tree, and *won*. Aging isn't just about the number of years we live, but how *vibrant* and *healthy* we feel during those years.

Think of your cells like rechargeable batteries. When we're young, they're fully charged and functioning at their best. But as we age, factors like stress, poor diet, toxins, and inactivity drain the battery.

The good news? **You can recharge it.** Longevity science shows that our bodies have incredible regenerative powers: if we provide the right conditions. Just like plugging in a smartphone keeps it running smoothly, optimizing nutrition, sleep, movement, and stress management keeps your cells "charged" for decades to come.

Imagine waking up at 80 years old feeling stronger, sharper, and more energetic than you did at 50. This isn't science fiction: it's the power of longevity science.

The choice is yours: Will you follow the outdated path of decline, or will you take action now to create a future filled with strength, clarity, and vitality? **Aging isn't a passive process**; it's something you can actively influence every day.

The healthcare industry doesn't promote longevity: it promotes chronic disease.

- **Medications for high blood pressure, diabetes, and cholesterol are billion-dollar industries**. But root-cause interventions like diet, fasting, and strength training **get no funding** because they don't generate ongoing revenue. (JAMA, 2020)

- **The average American senior takes over 5 prescription medications daily**, yet many of these diseases are preventable through lifestyle changes. (CDC, 2020)

- **Aging research is often funded by pharmaceutical companies**, not to extend health span, but to sell more drugs. (JAMA IM, 2019)

| Conventional Approach | Root-Cause Approach |
|---|---|
| Accept decline as "normal" | Take proactive steps to slow cellular aging |
| Treat diseases with medications | Prevent disease through diet, fasting, and exercise |
| Focus on lifespan (years lived) | Focus on health span (quality of life in those years) |
| Rely on surgeries and pharmaceuticals | Optimize hormones, mitochondria, and inflammation |
| View aging as irreversible | View aging as malleable and within your control |

**The reality?** The true path to longevity isn't found in a pill: it's found in daily choices that optimize your biology.

## Myths vs. Truths About Aging

| Myth | Truth |
|---|---|
| Aging is purely genetic. | Only 20% of aging is genetic; 80% is driven by lifestyle choices. Longevity is in your hands. |
| **Action Step:** Track your daily habits. Which ones are aging you faster? Which ones are supporting longevity? | |

| Strength training isn't important for aging. | Muscle is the strongest predictor of longevity. The more muscle you maintain, the longer and healthier you will live. |
|---|---|
| **Action Step:** Start resistance training 2-3 times per week, even bodyweight exercises count. ||

| Eating less and moving more is the key to longevity. | Nutrient timing (when you eat) is just as important as what you eat. Fasting activates autophagy, the body's cellular repair process. |
|---|---|
| **Action Step:** Try intermittent fasting (12 to 16 hour fasting window) and focus on nutrient-dense meals. ||

# The Longevity Code: How to Live Longer and Feel Younger

Did you know the world's longest-lived people don't just add years to their life? They add life to their years. In **Blue Zones**, regions known globally for extraordinary longevity and the highest concentrations of centenarians, there are people living healthily to 100 years or older. Aging isn't about decline; it's about sustained energy, sharp minds, and vibrant health.

Meanwhile, in much of the modern world, aging is associated with disease, fatigue, and memory loss. But what if we could change that?

What if aging didn't mean slowing down but instead meant maintaining strength, mental clarity, and vitality for decades longer? Science now shows that with the right lifestyle choices, we *can* slow, and even *reverse*, the aging process.

Science now shows that aging is not just about years lived but about biological health, and much of it is within our control. In this chapter, we will explore:

- The **root causes** of aging and how to slow them down.
- The **role of cellular repair, telomeres, and mitochondria** in longevity.
- **Breakthrough strategies related to longevity**, including fasting, exercise, nutrition, and mindset, that can help you age gracefully.
- A **30-day longevity plan** to implement anti-aging habits today.

## The Science of Aging: What Speeds It Up and How to Slow It Down

Aging is influenced by a combination of genetics and lifestyle factors. Although we can't alter our DNA, we have significant control over key factors that accelerate premature aging:

**Chronic Inflammation:** Often termed *"inflammaging,"* chronic inflammation speeds aging at the cellular level, causing wrinkles, joint pain, cognitive decline, and chronic diseases.

## How to control it:

- Adopt an anti-inflammatory diet rich in vegetables, healthy fats, and omega-3 fatty acids

- Reduce processed foods and sugar intake

- Regularly engage in moderate exercise

- Practice stress management techniques like meditation or yoga

**Oxidative Stress:** An excess of free radicals leads to oxidative stress, damaging cells, DNA, and mitochondria, contributing to rapid aging.

## How to control it:

- Increase consumption of antioxidant-rich foods like berries, leafy greens, nuts, and spices such as turmeric and ginger

- Limit exposure to toxins and pollutants

- Avoid smoking

- Incorporate regular physical activity to boost antioxidant defenses

**Mitochondrial Decline:** Our mitochondria (often called the "powerhouses of the cells") lose efficiency with age, causing decreased energy, slower metabolism, and impaired cognitive function.

**How to control it:**

- Engage in regular aerobic exercise and strength training to enhance mitochondrial function

- Practice intermittent fasting

- Optimize sleep quality

- Consume mitochondrial-supportive nutrients such as Coenzyme Q10 (CoQ10), L-Carnitine, and magnesium

**Telomere Shortening:** Telomeres, the protective caps at the ends of DNA strands, naturally shorten as we age, but unhealthy lifestyle factors accelerate this process.

**How to control it:**

- Follow a nutrient-rich diet high in antioxidants

- Manage stress through mindfulness practices

- Prioritize adequate sleep

- Incorporate regular physical activity

Research published in *Nature Medicine* shows individuals who actively maintain an anti-inflammatory diet, engage in regular physical activity, and practice consistent stress management significantly slow the aging process, reduce their risk for chronic diseases, and maintain youthful energy and vitality well into their later years.

## The Key to Longevity: Cellular Repair and Telomere Health

Think of your body as a city. Over time, buildings wear down, roads develop cracks, and pollution accumulates. Without maintenance, the city slowly crumbles. But with regular repairs, efficient waste removal, and smart upgrades, it remains vibrant and functional for decades. Your body works the same way. It has built-in repair mechanisms (cellular renewal, detoxification, and regeneration) that keep you strong and resilient. Other examples of these repair mechanisms include:

# Telomeres: The Aging Clock

Telomeres are like the protective tips on shoelaces, preventing DNA from unraveling. As they shorten over time, cells lose their ability to function properly, accelerating aging and disease. The key to a longer, healthier life is preserving telomere length. Some ways to do that include:

- **Reducing chronic stress:** Meditation, gratitude, deep breathing
- **Exercising regularly:** A mix of cardio and strength training
- **Consuming antioxidant-rich foods:** Berries, green tea, nuts

# Autophagy: The Body's Self-Cleaning Process

Autophagy is your body's natural cleanup process, clearing out damaged cells and making way for new, healthy ones. Think of it as a deep detox at the cellular level: essential for slowing aging, reducing inflammation, and protecting against disease. Some ways to activate and enhance autophagy include:

- **Intermittent fasting:** Fasting for 12 to 16 hours triggers autophagy
- **Cold exposure**: Ice baths, cryotherapy

- **Polyphenol-rich foods**: Dark chocolate, turmeric, blueberries

## The Ultimate Anti-Aging Toolkit: Nutrition, Supplements, and Lifestyle

The key to longevity isn't just in your genes: it's in your daily choices. This anti-aging toolkit combines science-backed nutrition, targeted supplements, and lifestyle strategies to slow aging at the cellular level, boost energy, and enhance overall vitality.

**1. Eat for Longevity:**

- **Fatty Fish**: Omega-3s reduce inflammation and protect the brain.
- **Leafy Greens**: Spinach, kale, and arugula fight oxidative stress.
- **Berries**: Rich in polyphenols that slow aging.
- **Avocados & Nuts**: Healthy fats that support cell repair.
- **Turmeric**: A powerhouse for inflammation control.

**2. Longevity-Boosting Supplements:**

- **Resveratrol**: Found in red wine, mimics the effects of fasting.

- **NAD+ Boosters (NMN or NR)**: Enhance DNA repair and energy.
- **Magnesium**: Critical for stress reduction and sleep quality.

## 3. Move to Stay Young:

- **Strength Training**: Maintains muscle mass and metabolic health.
- **Daily Walking**: Improves circulation and brain function.
- **HIIT Workouts**: Boosts mitochondrial efficiency.

## 4. Biohacking for Longevity:

- **Wearables**: Use an **Oura Ring** or **CGM** to track health markers.
- **Cold Therapy**: Stimulates autophagy and fat-burning.
- **Sunlight & Red-Light Therapy**: Supports mitochondria and skin health.

*Any nutritional, supplement or technology recommendations are intended to support general wellness and are not meant to diagnose, treat, or prevent any disease. Consult your healthcare provider before starting any diet or supplement program.

# Your 30-Day Action Plan: Longevity Reset

Aging *is* a choice, and in today's modern world we can control aging more than ever before. Advances in longevity research reveal that factors like nutrition, movement, sleep, stress management, and targeted therapies can slow biological aging, enhance cellular repair, and extend both lifespan and healthspan. Try following this step-by-step, week-by-week plan to begin having control over your rate of aging:

## WEEK 1: Nutrition & Fasting

- Cut out processed foods and sugar.
- Start intermittent fasting (12 hours).
- Increase antioxidants and omega-3s.

## WEEK 2: Movement & Recovery

- Strength train **2 to 3 times per week**.
- Walk **10,000+ steps daily**.
- Prioritize deep sleep (limit blue light exposure).

## WEEK 3: Stress & Detox

- Try **meditation, deep breathing,** or **gratitude journaling**.

- Drink **more water** and add electrolytes.
- Reduce inflammation with sauna or cold therapy.

**WEEK 4: Biohacking & Optimization**

- Track health with a wearable (sleep, HRV, glucose).
- Experiment with **time-restricted eating (16:8 fasting).**
- Engage in **lifelong learning to stimulate the brain.**

I have seen that by incorporating simple, science-backed habits, you can extend your health span, enhance energy, and maintain vitality for decades. Aging does *not* have to mean decline. Science proves that your habits today determine your quality-of-life decades from now. Will you accept the standard aging model, or will you take control and create a future of strength, vitality, and mental clarity?

## Next Up

In **Chapter 13**, we'll explore the truth about alcohol's impact on health and how to build a healthier relationship with drinking.

# Chapter 13:

# Alcohol's Hidden Toll: What Drinking Really Costs Your Health

# Did You Know? Alcohol Kills More People Than All Drugs Combined

**Alcohol is responsible for over 3 million deaths worldwide each year: more than all illicit drugs combined** (*World Health Organization, 2022*).

At 42, Lisa felt drained. Her energy was low, her weight kept creeping up, and her anxiety was through the roof. She didn't consider herself a "heavy drinker," but a few glasses of wine each evening had become her routine. Then, a routine blood test revealed the truth: **fatty liver, elevated blood sugar, and prediabetes**. She was stunned. She wasn't overweight, didn't binge drink, and didn't "feel" sick. Yet, alcohol had been silently harming her body. Determined to take control, Lisa quit drinking for 90 days.

The transformation was *undeniable*: her energy returned, brain fog lifted, cravings subsided, liver function improved, and anxiety melted away. It wasn't a coincidence. It was *science*. Alcohol had been the

Achilles heel in her health struggles. Lisa never looked back, and today, she feels stronger, clearer, and more in control than ever before.

Alcohol is like a deceptive credit card with hidden fees. At first, it feels like an easy indulgence: an occasional drink to unwind, celebrate, or socialize. But just like swiping a credit card without thinking, the balance starts to build. Over time, interest accrues in ways you don't immediately notice: liver damage, inflammation, disrupted sleep, weight gain, and a higher risk of disease. Your body keeps a meticulous account, and eventually, the bill comes due: often at a **much higher cost** than expected.

The problem? Most people don't realize how much alcohol is silently draining their health until it's too late. The solution isn't a temporary detox or cutting back for a month: it's turning off the faucet. The good news? Unlike financial debt, your body has the remarkable ability to repair itself when given the right conditions. The *sooner* you take control, the more *freedom* you reclaim.

We live in a society where alcohol is normalized, celebrated, and even encouraged. It's the centerpiece of social gatherings, business meetings, and stress relief. But what if the very thing marketed as a "relaxant" is actually accelerating chronic disease, mental decline, and metabolic dysfunction? Alcohol isn't just a temporary indulgence: it has **lasting consequences** on the brain, liver, heart, and gut. This chapter exposes the truth about alcohol's impact, debunks myths, and empowers you to *rethink* your relationship with drinking.

The alcohol industry makes billions promoting "moderation" while the healthcare system struggles from alcohol-induced disease.

- Medications for **liver disease, high blood pressure, and depression** are booming industries.

- **Alcohol-related cancers are on the rise**, but few doctors talk about it.

- **Rehab centers, detox programs, and antidepressant prescriptions** increase as alcohol dependency grows.

| Conventional Approach | Root-Cause Approach |
|---|---|
| "Drink in moderation; it's fine!" | "Even moderate drinking has risks; be mindful." |
| Medication for anxiety, liver disease, and inflammation | Address the root cause: remove alcohol and heal naturally |
| Ignore gut health and metabolism | Prioritize liver detox, gut microbiome balance, and hydration |

| | |
|---|---|
| Assume alcohol is necessary for socializing | Learn to enjoy social events without alcohol dependence |

**What would happen if you gave your body 30 days without alcohol?** Will you challenge yourself to rethink your relationship with alcohol and discover what life could feel like without it?

## Myths vs. Truths About Alcohol

| Myth | Truth |
|---|---|
| Alcohol helps you relax and sleep. | Alcohol disrupts deep sleep cycles, leaving you groggy and exhausted. |
| **Action Step:** Try magnesium, herbal tea, or deep breathing instead of alcohol to unwind. | |

| | |
|---|---|
| Red wine is good for your heart. | While red wine contains resveratrol, an antioxidant that can help reduce oxidative stress, support cardiovascular health, improve insulin sensitivity, and potentially slow aging by activating proteins called sirtuins. However, you'd need to drink dozens of bottles to get meaningful benefits, without the toxic side effects. |

| | |
|---|---|
| **Action Step:** Get antioxidants from berries, dark chocolate, and green tea, without the alcohol. | |

| | |
|---|---|
| Alcohol is only harmful if you drink too much | Even moderate alcohol consumption increases the risk of cancer, heart disease, and metabolic dysfunction. |
| **Action Step:** Challenge yourself to 30 days alcohol-free and experience the health transformation. | |

## The Hidden Cost of Alcohol: Chronic Disease and Economic Impact

Alcohol consumption comes with a staggering economic toll in the United States, **costing approximately $249 billion annually**, a figure that has been steadily increasing over the past decade according to the CDC. These costs are not just limited to healthcare expenses, but also include lost workplace productivity, motor vehicle accidents, and criminal justice expenditures.

Even more alarming is alcohol's role in fueling the escalating costs of chronic diseases, such as **liver disease, diabetes, cardiovascular disease,** and **certain cancers**. The American Journal of Preventive Medicine highlights that nearly half of alcohol-related healthcare expenditures, amounting to billions of dollars every year, stem directly from chronic conditions exacerbated by drinking.

As alcohol consumption continues to rise in the U.S., the hidden financial and health costs are becoming harder to ignore, urging individuals and healthcare policymakers alike to re-evaluate alcohol's accepted place in daily life.

## How Alcohol Affects Your Body

Alcohol is more than just empty calories: it directly interferes with critical bodily functions. A meta-analysis in *The Lancet* concluded that no amount of alcohol is truly safe, challenging the belief that moderate drinking is beneficial. Here are just a few of the ways that alcohol is negatively impacting your health, mind, and life:

- **Liver Damage & Detox Disruption**: Excessive drinking overwhelms the liver, leading to fatty liver disease, inflammation, and eventual cirrhosis.

- **Gut Microbiome Imbalance**: Alcohol disrupts gut bacteria, contributing to leaky gut, poor digestion, and immune dysfunction.

- **Increased Cancer Risk**: The World Health Organization classifies alcohol as a Group 1 carcinogen, linked to cancers of the liver, breast, esophagus, and colon.

- **Blood Sugar Spikes & Insulin Resistance**: Chronic alcohol use contributes to metabolic dysfunction, increasing the risk of Type 2 diabetes.

- **Neurological Damage**: Long-term alcohol consumption alters brain chemistry, affecting memory, cognitive function, and emotional regulation.

## How to Minimize the Damage & Take Control

If you drink, taking steps to mitigate harm is crucial. By being mindful of how much and how often you drink, and making conscious efforts to prioritize hydration, balanced nutrition, and overall wellness, you can minimize the negative impact alcohol has on your body. Some other helpful tips to minimize damage include:

1. **Follow the 2:1 Rule**: For every alcoholic drink, drink two glasses of water to support detoxification.
2. **Choose Lower-Toxin Alcohols**: Clear liquors (vodka, tequila) contain fewer additives than wine or beer.

3. **Support Liver Detox**: Milk thistle, glutathione, and turmeric help protect liver function.

4. **Set Alcohol-Free Days**: Having at least 3 to 4 alcohol-free days per week allows the body to recover.

5. **Assess Your Relationship with Alcohol**: Track your intake and recognize any emotional or habitual dependencies.

6. **Explore Alternatives**: Mocktails, adaptogenic drinks, and non-alcoholic spirits provide a social drinking experience without the health risks.

# Your 30-Day Action Plan: Alcohol Reset

When it comes to alcohol consumption, do your best to make wise choices. Be mindful of how much you drink and how often, and consider how it affects your physical and mental well-being. Remember, the goal is not just to limit harm but to create a lifestyle where your body and mind thrive, both now and in the long term. Consider implementing this step-by-step, week-by-week action plan to start your alcohol-free life today:

### WEEK 1: Reduce Alcohol & Hydrate More
- Cut your alcohol intake in half.
- Drink two glasses of water for every alcoholic drink.

### WEEK 2: Swap Alcohol for Healthier Alternatives
- Try **herbal teas, sparkling water, or adaptogenic drinks** instead of alcohol.
- Journal your moods to see how you feel without alcohol.

### WEEK 3: Go Alcohol-Free for 7 Days
- Remove alcohol completely and track your **energy, sleep, and cravings.**
- Prioritize **liver-supporting foods** like turmeric, cruciferous veggies, and lemon water.

**WEEK 4: Reintroduce Mindfully (or Stay Alcohol-Free!)**

- If reintroducing alcohol, **stick to small amounts and high-quality choices.**
- If staying alcohol-free, celebrate your **improved health, clarity, and energy.**

**Action Step:** Start your alcohol reset **today.**

While alcohol is socially accepted, it's one of the biggest silent contributors to chronic disease. Understanding its effects allows you to make empowered choices. Whether you reduce your intake, quit entirely, or simply drink more mindfully, you have the power to reclaim your health. What if your anxiety disappeared? What if your metabolism improved? What if you woke up every day feeling amazing?

The answer is within your reach. The choice is yours.

## Next Up

In **Chapter 14**, we'll focus on creating a personalized roadmap to sustain these lifelong health habits.

# PART III:
# Lasting Health – Your Blueprint for Lifelong Wellness

# Chapter 14:

# Mind Over Disease: Harnessing the Mind-Body Connection

Did You Know? Chronic Stress Can Take 10+ Years Off Your Life

**Studies show that chronic stress accelerates aging at the cellular level, shortening telomeres (the protective caps on our DNA) by up to 10 years** (*Proceedings of the National Academy of Sciences*).

We often view stress and mental health as separate from physical health, but research reveals that chronic stress, anxiety, and trauma can directly lead to inflammation, metabolic dysfunction, and even autoimmune disorders. Your mental state doesn't *just* influence your emotions: it impacts your body's functioning at a cellular level.

For years, David battled rheumatoid arthritis, chronic fatigue, and severe digestive issues. His doctors prescribed anti-inflammatory drugs, painkillers, and steroids, but his condition only worsened. One day, while reading about the connection between trauma and chronic disease, David realized something significant: his health had started to decline after a devastating personal loss. Determined to heal, he began meditating, practicing deep breathing, and working with a therapist to address unresolved emotions. The results? Within six months, his pain decreased by 70%, he reduced his medications, and his energy returned. His gut health improved, and inflammation markers dropped. **David's transformation wasn't a coincidence**; it was the power of mental healing, unlocking his body's ability to repair itself.

Your mind and body are like the conductor and the orchestra. The mind, as the conductor, sets the rhythm, harmony, and energy that guide every instrument, the body's organs, systems, and functions. When the conductor is calm and in sync, the orchestra plays a beautiful symphony of health, balance, and vitality. But when the conductor is overwhelmed, stressed, or out of sync, the music becomes chaotic: some instruments play too loudly, others too softly, and the entire performance suffers. This disharmony shows up as chronic inflammation, weakened immunity, and disease. True wellness is about tuning the mind so the body can perform. When we calm the conductor, through mindfulness, stress reduction, and emotional balance, the whole orchestra comes back into harmony, creating a life filled with health, energy, and resilience.

**Imagine** living free from chronic stress, waking up energized, and feeling emotionally lighter. **Imagine** taking control of your mental well-being and unlocking a healthier, more vibrant body. Your thoughts, emotions, and stress levels shape your physical health. Will you take the next step toward healing?

## The Science of Stress & Disease

A study in *The Lancet Psychiatry* found that people with severe mental distress had a **32% higher risk** of developing chronic disease. The takeaway? Your mind isn't separate from your body; it controls your health at a cellular level.

- **Chronic Stress & Inflammation**: Stress raises cortisol, which triggers inflammation and contributes to heart disease, obesity, and neurodegeneration.

- **Trauma & Autoimmune Disorders**: Studies show that unresolved trauma increases the risk of lupus, multiple sclerosis, and rheumatoid arthritis.

- **Anxiety, Depression & Metabolic Health**: Mental distress disrupts insulin function, blood pressure, and digestion, increasing disease risk.

The healthcare system relies on prescribing antidepressants, anti-anxiety meds, and painkillers, without addressing the root cause.

| Conventional Approach | Root-Cause Approach |
|---|---|
| Prescribe antidepressants for stress and anxiety | Identify and heal the root cause of stress |
| Recommend painkillers for chronic pain | Use mind-body techniques to reduce pain naturally |
| Ignore the link between trauma and physical illness | Address trauma and emotional health to improve overall wellness |
| Overlook the role of gut health in mental illness | Heal the gut microbiome to restore mood balance |

**The truth?** Chronic disease and mental illness feed each other in a cycle, and the healthcare system continues to struggle. Instead of addressing stress, trauma, and gut-brain imbalances, the system focuses on symptom suppression, leading to lifelong medication dependency.

# Myths vs. Truths About Mental Health & Chronic Disease

| Myth | Truth |
|------|-------|
| Mental health only affects emotions, not physical health. | Chronic stress disrupts hormones, gut health, and immune function, leading to real disease. |
| **Action Step:** Start a daily stress-reducing habit (meditation, deep breathing, nature walks). | |

| | |
|------|-------|
| If a chronic disease is genetic, mental health won't change the outcome. | Epigenetics proves that stress reduction and mental resilience can "turn off" disease-triggering genes. |
| **Action Step:** Try mindfulness exercises to reprogram your brain for healing. | |

| | |
|------|-------|
| Trauma is purely psychological and doesn't affect the body. | Unresolved trauma increases inflammation, weakens immunity, and raises disease risk. |
| **Action Step:** Consider therapy, Eye Movement Desensitization and Reprocessing **(EMDR)** a psychotherapy technique designed to help individuals heal from emotional distress and trauma, or journaling to process past trauma. | |

# The Hidden Link: How Mental Health Influences Chronic Disease

For decades, chronic diseases like diabetes, heart disease, and autoimmune disorders have been viewed primarily through the lens of physical health. However, research now confirms that mental health is a major player in disease progression and recovery. The connection is clear: treating the mind is just as important as treating the body. Here are some examples of how mental and physical health coincide:

- **Chronic Stress & Inflammation**: Stress triggers the release of cortisol, the body's primary stress hormone. While short-term cortisol spikes are protective, chronic elevation leads to systemic inflammation, a known driver of heart disease, obesity, and even neurodegeneration.

- **Trauma & Autoimmune Disorders**: Studies in *The Journal of Psychosomatic Research* have shown that unresolved trauma increases the risk of autoimmune diseases like lupus, rheumatoid arthritis, and multiple sclerosis.

- **Anxiety, Depression, and Metabolic Health**: Mental health disorders are linked to poor metabolic function. Depression and anxiety increase insulin resistance, elevate blood pressure, and impair digestion, leading to a higher risk of diabetes and cardiovascular disease.

## The Power of Neuroplasticity: Rewiring the Brain for Healing

Neuroplasticity is the brain's ability to rewire itself in response to new experiences, thoughts, and behaviors. This means that healing from chronic disease isn't just about medication and diet; it's also about retraining the brain.

**How Neuroplasticity Supports Healing:**

- **Reduces Stress Response**: Mindfulness, meditation, and breathwork train the brain to lower stress hormones, reducing inflammation.

- **Improves Pain Perception**: Chronic pain conditions like fibromyalgia respond to neuroplasticity-based interventions such as cognitive behavioral therapy (CBT) and movement-based therapies like yoga.

- **Boosts Immune Function**: A study from *Psychoneuroendocrinology* found that mindfulness-based practices increase T-cell activity, strengthening immune resilience.

Harnessing neuroplasticity through intentional mental practices can create profound changes in physical health. Here are some effective practices to consider:

**Mindfulness and Meditation:** Regular meditation practice strengthens neural pathways involved in emotional regulation, stress reduction, and pain management. Studies show mindfulness can lower inflammation, reduce cortisol levels, and improve immune system responses, leading to fewer illnesses and faster healing.

**Visualization and Mental Imagery:** Athletes and rehabilitation patients use visualization to enhance performance and recovery. By repeatedly visualizing successful movements, the brain creates stronger neural pathways, helping muscles recover faster and improving coordination and strength.

**Cognitive Behavioral Therapy (CBT):** CBT actively retrains thought patterns from negative, stress-inducing beliefs to more positive, constructive ones. This shift in thinking physically reduces the stress response, decreasing inflammation and supporting cardiovascular health.

**Positive Affirmations and Gratitude Practices:** Regularly practicing gratitude and repeating positive affirmations can reshape neural networks associated with happiness, optimism, and emotional resilience, thereby lowering blood pressure, improving heart health, and boosting overall immune function.

**Yoga and Tai Chi:** These mind-body practices combine movement with breathwork and meditation, rewiring the brain for improved balance, reduced pain perception, and increased flexibility. Clinical evidence demonstrates yoga and tai chi can relieve chronic pain, decrease inflammation, and boost immunity.

## How to Strengthen the Mind-Body Connection for Chronic Disease Healing

To optimize both mental and physical health in order to strengthen your body and mind against chronic disease, consider these science-backed strategies:

**Reduce Chronic Stress:**
- Practice **deep breathing** (4-7-8 method) to lower cortisol.
- Engage in **meditation or mindfulness** for at least 10 minutes per day.
- Spend time in nature, shown to reduce stress markers by 30%.

**Heal Unresolved Trauma:**
- Consider EMDR therapy (Eye Movement Desensitization and Reprocessing) for past trauma.

- Journaling can help reprocess painful experiences.
- Seek professional support if needed; mental health therapy has profound physical health benefits.

**Adopt a Resilient Mindset:**
- **Gratitude practice**: Writing down three things you're grateful for daily has been shown to improve immune function.
- **Cognitive Reframing**: Reinterpreting negative events in a neutral or positive light strengthens mental resilience and lowers stress hormones.

**Improve Sleep for Brain Detoxification:**
- Aim for 7 to 9 hours of high-quality sleep to allow the glymphatic system to remove toxins from the brain.
- Reduce blue light exposure 2 hours before bed.
- Create a bedtime routine to signal the brain it's time to rest.

**Engage in Movement & Breathwork:**
- **Yoga & Tai Chi**: These have been proven to reduce stress, lower inflammation, and enhance neuroplasticity.
- **Box Breathing**: A technique used by Navy SEALs, box breathing calms the nervous system and improves focus.

# Your 30-Day Action Plan: Mental Health Reset

Mental health is often seen as separate from physical health, but the truth is, they are deeply intertwined. Stress, trauma, and emotional well-being play a critical role in chronic disease, influencing everything from inflammation to immune function. Emerging research in neuroplasticity reveals that the brain and body are capable of remarkable healing when given the right tools. Below is a step-by-step, week-by-week action plan to begin prioritizing your mental health today:

## WEEK 1: Implement Daily Stress-Reduction Techniques
- Meditate or deep breathe for 5 to 10 minutes each day.
- Reduce screen time before bed for better sleep.

## WEEK 2: Heal Unresolved Trauma
- Try journaling or therapy to process past experiences.
- Engage in self-care practices that bring emotional relief.

## WEEK 3: Strengthen Your Mind-Body Connection
- Incorporate yoga, tai chi, or mindful movement.
- Spend time in nature to reduce stress markers.

## WEEK 4: Build Resilience & Gratitude
- Write 3 things you're grateful for daily.

- Reframe negative thoughts using cognitive behavioral techniques.

**Action Step:** Choose one **mind-body healing habit** to start today!

The future of medicine is integrative, acknowledging that mental and physical health are one and the same. I have seen over the years that by addressing emotional well-being, reducing chronic stress, and harnessing neuroplasticity, we can significantly lower disease risk, accelerate healing, and build a more resilient body. **Your mind is the most powerful tool for healing.** Your thoughts can trigger stress, or promote peace. Your emotions can fuel disease, or drive recovery. Your mindset can keep you stuck, or set you free. **You are not powerless.** You can rewire your brain, regulate your emotions, and take control of your health.

## Next Up

In **Chapter 15**, we'll explore the power of fasting and autophagy, a revolutionary tool for cellular regeneration and disease prevention.

# Chapter 15:

# Fasting for Longevity: How Autophagy Renews Your Body

## Did You Know? Fasting Can Extend Your Life and Reduce Disease Risk

**A groundbreaking study in the New England Journal of Medicine found that fasting can increase lifespan by up to 30%, reduce the risk of cancer, and enhance cognitive function.**

For centuries, fasting has been used in spiritual, cultural, and medical practices, but today, science is proving its profound impact on cellular regeneration, metabolism, and disease prevention. **The reality?** Fasting is not starvation; it's a tool for unlocking the body's natural healing abilities.

For years, Maria battled obesity, insulin resistance, and brain fog. Despite following traditional dieting advice, eating small meals every few hours, her weight kept increasing, and her blood sugar worsened. At 50, her doctor warned she was heading toward Type 2 diabetes. Feeling defeated, Maria discovered intermittent fasting and committed to a 16:8 fasting schedule (fasting for 16 hours and eating within an 8-hour window). In just a few months, she experienced 40 pounds of weight loss without starving herself, improved mental clarity and energy, and reversed insulin resistance with stabilized blood sugar levels. Maria's transformation wasn't a fluke; **science supported it**. Fasting helped reset her metabolism and activated autophagy, allowing her body to **heal naturally**.

Think of your body like a self-cleaning oven. When you're constantly eating, your body doesn't have the opportunity to clear out waste and toxins. But when you fast, your body activates autophagy, its natural cleaning system, to eliminate damaged cells, clear toxins, and rejuvenate itself. Fasting triggers this deep-cleaning mode, allowing your body to reset and improve long-term health.

## Unlock the Power of Fasting

Imagine waking up with more energy, clearer thinking, and a body that effortlessly burns fat. Picture harnessing your body's natural ability to heal and regenerate. Fasting isn't just a temporary diet; it's a powerful, life-changing approach to reclaim your health. The real question is: Are you ready to embrace it?

Fasting is free, but medications are not. Big Pharma rakes in billions from treating conditions like diabetes, obesity, and heart disease, yet rarely promotes fasting, a natural solution proven to reverse these issues. Instead of teaching people how to reverse disease through metabolic healing, the healthcare system pushes lifelong prescriptions and expensive treatments. It's time to take control of your health, without relying on a system that profits from keeping you sick.

| Conventional Approach | Root-Cause Approach |
|---|---|
| Eat every few hours to "boost metabolism" | Fasting improves insulin sensitivity and burns fat naturally |
| Prescribe medications for diabetes and obesity | Use fasting to reverse insulin resistance |
| Focus on calorie restriction | Focus on hormonal balance and metabolic flexibility |
| Fear fasting, thinking it leads to starvation | Embrace fasting as a tool for cellular repair and longevity |

**The truth?** Fasting isn't extreme; it's what our bodies were designed to do.

## Myths vs. Truths About Fasting

| Myth | Truth |
|---|---|
| Fasting causes muscle loss. | Fasting increases growth hormone, which preserves muscle. |
| **Action Step:** Incorporate strength training during fasting to maintain muscle mass. | |

| Skipping meals slows metabolism. | Research shows short-term fasting boosts metabolic rate by up to 14%. |
|---|---|
| **Action Step:** Start with **a** 12-hour fast and gradually increase to 16 hours. | |

| Fasting makes you tired and weak. | Once adapted, fasting stabilizes energy and improves mental clarity. |
|---|---|
| **Action Step:** Drink electrolytes and stay hydrated to prevent fatigue. | |

# The Science of Fasting: Why It's a Game-Changer for Health

Fasting is the intentional practice of abstaining from food for a set period of time, allowing the body a chance to transition from digestion to deep repair mode. Research shows that fasting improves insulin sensitivity, lowers inflammation, sharpens brain function, and activates autophagy.

**What happens when you fast?**

- **At 12 hours:** Insulin levels drop, allowing the body to burn stored fat for energy.

- **At 16 hours:** Autophagy begins, clearing out damaged cells and regenerating healthier ones.

- **At 24 hours:** Growth hormone surges, preserving muscle mass and supporting cellular repair.

- **At 48-72 hours:** Stem cell production increases, boosting immune function and longevity.

A study published in *Cell Metabolism* revealed that intermittent fasting significantly improves mitochondrial function, the energy-producing centers of our cells. By enhancing mitochondrial efficiency, fasting helps reduce oxidative stress: one of the key drivers of aging and disease. Researchers also found that intermittent fasting lowers the risk of chronic conditions such as Type 2 diabetes, Alzheimer's disease, and heart disease by improving metabolic health, reducing inflammation, and supporting cellular repair processes.

## Autophagy: Your Body's Natural Detox Mechanism

Autophagy, which translates to "self-eating," is the body's natural process of cleaning out damaged cells, misfolded proteins, and cellular debris, reducing the accumulation of waste that leads to aging and disease.

**Benefits of autophagy include:**

- **Clearing damaged cells** to prevent diseases like cancer and neurodegeneration.

- **Improving insulin sensitivity**, reducing the risk of diabetes.

- **Enhancing brain function** by protecting neurons from oxidative stress.

- **Boosting longevity** by slowing the biological aging process.

A study published in *Nature* found that activating autophagy through fasting is essential for **cellular rejuvenation, strengthening the immune system, and extending lifespan**. By clearing out damaged cells and recycling their components, autophagy helps protect against age-related diseases, enhances metabolic efficiency, and supports overall health. This research highlights fasting as a powerful tool for promoting longevity and disease prevention.

# Types of Fasting & How to Choose the Right One

There are several fasting methods, each offering distinct benefits depending on your health goals:

1. **Intermittent Fasting (16:8)**: Fast for 16 hours, eat within an 8-hour window.
   - Great for beginners, improves metabolic health.

2. **Time-Restricted Eating (TRE)**: Eat only during a set window (e.g., 10 am - 6 pm).
   - Supports circadian rhythm and digestion.

3. **One-Meal-A-Day (OMAD)**: Eating one large meal per day.
   - Simplifies nutrition, enhances fat loss.

4. **24-48 Hour Fasting**: No food for one to two full days.
   - Promotes deep autophagy and immune system reset.

5. **Extended Fasting (3-5 days)**: Long fasts to boost stem cell production and longevity.
   - **Not** recommended for beginners but beneficial for cellular repair.

## How to Fast Safely: A Step-by-Step Guide

No matter what fasting method you choose, there are some general rules you should follow in order to fast both safety and effectively:

**Step 1: Choose Your Fasting Window**: Start with a 12-hour fast and gradually extend.

**Step 2: Prioritize Hydration**: Drink water, herbal teas, and electrolytes.

**Step 3: Eat Nutrient-Dense Meals**: Break your fast with whole foods rich in protein, fiber, and healthy fats.

**Step 4: Avoid Processed Foods**: Stick to real, whole foods to maximize benefits.

**Step 5: Listen to Your Body**: If feeling weak or overly fatigued, adjust your fasting duration.

## Who Should Be Cautious with Fasting?

While fasting offers numerous health benefits, it may not be suitable for everyone. Certain individuals should consult a healthcare provider before attempting extended fasts, including:

- **Pregnant or breastfeeding women**
- **People with a history of eating disorders**
- **Individuals with low blood sugar or adrenal issues**
- **Those on medications that require food intake**

# Your 30-Day Action Plan: Fasting Reset

Fasting is not a new concept; it has been practiced for centuries in various cultures for spiritual, mental, and physical benefits. But modern science has confirmed that fasting does more than just promote discipline; it activates a powerful cellular repair process called **autophagy**, which helps extend lifespan, improve metabolic health, and reverse chronic disease. If you think fasting might be right for you, try following this step-by-step, week-by-week action plan for the first month:

**WEEK 1:** Try a 12-hour fasting window (e.g., 8 PM - 8 AM).

**WEEK 2:** Increase to a 14-16 hour fast (e.g., 6 PM - 10 AM).

**WEEK 3:** Experiment with a 24-hour fast once per week.

**WEEK 4:** Listen to your body, mix up fasting lengths, and track your progress.

**Action Step:** Start with **a simple 12-hour fast today.** Small changes lead to big results.

Fasting is not just about weight loss; it's about cellular repair, longevity, and disease prevention. I have seen firsthand that by incorporating fasting into your routine, you can enhance brain function, balance metabolism, and unlock the body's natural healing potential. Are *you* ready to reclaim your health and unlock the power of fasting?

## Next Up

In **Chapter 16**, we'll explore the importance of peptides, and how they can help the body send signals, heal tissues, and support vital functions like growth and immunity.

# Chapter 16:

# Peptides Unlocked: The Body's Secret Code for Accelerated Healing and Recovery

Did You Know? Peptides May Support the Body's Natural Healing Potential

**More than 133 million Americans suffer from chronic illnesses, conditions that conventional medicine often struggles to heal. But what if the keys to unlocking deep, lasting healing already exist within your body, waiting to be activated? The latest groundbreaking research points toward a promising solution: peptides.**

## Peptides 101: Your Body's Natural Messengers

Peptides are short chains of amino acids (the fundamental building blocks of proteins) that act as messengers within your body. Think of them as tiny couriers, rapidly delivering instructions to cells, tissues, and organs, guiding them how to repair, rebuild, and rejuvenate. Since peptides naturally occur in the body, **they play a crucial role in healing, growth, and immune function.**

What makes peptides especially powerful is their precision. Unlike broad, generalized treatments, **peptides target specific tissues and functions,** supporting natural and effective healing responses.

## Peptides and Chronic Disease: What Science Says

Recent studies in prestigious journals like Nature, Cell, and the Journal of Clinical Investigation highlight the promising potential of peptides to combat and reverse chronic diseases by reducing inflammation, promoting tissue repair, boosting metabolism, and strengthening the immune system.

Conventional medicine has been slow to embrace peptides, often prioritizing pharmaceuticals over these natural healing agents, despite growing evidence of their effectiveness in restoring health and vitality.

While peptides are not intended to replace pharmaceutical interventions, they may complement conventional medicine by working in harmony with the body's natural repair systems.

**Here's why peptides are gaining traction in the world of health optimization:**

- **Reduced Inflammation:** Peptides like BPC-157 and TB-500 actively reduce inflammation and accelerate the repair of tissues, bones, and muscles.

- **Improved Joint and Bone Health:** Collagen peptides boost cartilage strength, reduce joint pain, and support bone density.

- **Enhanced Muscle Growth and Recovery:** Peptides like IGF-1 LR3 and Growth Hormone-Releasing Peptides (GHRPs) naturally boost your body's production of growth hormone, dramatically improving muscle repair, fat loss, and metabolic health.

- **Boosted Immunity and Infection Defense:** Antimicrobial peptides (AMPs) protect against harmful bacteria and viruses, bolstering the immune system at a fundamental level.

## Meet the Peptide Powerhouses

Here's a closer look at some powerful peptides you can integrate into your healing journey:

- **BPC-157**: Naturally found in your stomach, this peptide promotes rapid healing of tissues, tendons, ligaments, and bones. It's ideal for recovery after injuries or chronic inflammation.

- **TB-500**: This peptide stimulates new tissue growth, increases flexibility, and reduces pain and inflammation. It's great for supporting faster healing after strenuous exercise or injuries.

- **Collagen Peptides**: These hydrolyzed proteins nourish joints, strengthen hair and skin, and support muscle recovery and gut health.

- **Growth Hormone-Releasing Peptides (GHRPs)**: GHRPs naturally stimulate your body's growth hormone production, aiding fat loss, muscle growth, improved sleep, and anti-aging benefits.

- **IGF-1 LR3**: This peptide boosts muscle protein synthesis, supporting lean muscle development, metabolism, and recovery.

- **Antimicrobial Peptides (AMPs)**: These peptides strengthen immune responses by directly combating pathogens, keeping you resilient against infections

- **PT-141 (Bremelanotide)** is a melanocortin receptor agonist originally studied for sexual dysfunction. It acts on the central nervous system, potentially enhancing arousal, energy, and mood by modulating key neurochemical pathways in the brain.

You stand at the edge of transformation, with your body's untapped potential ready to awaken. Just as a symphony conductor guides each note into harmony, peptides signal your cells to heal and regenerate. Today, you have the opportunity to take control: to reclaim your health, unlock your body's natural power, and rewrite your wellness story.

# Myths vs. Truths About Peptides

| Myth | Truth |
|---|---|
| Peptides are unnatural chemicals or steroids. | Peptides are naturally occurring short chains of amino acids; your body already produces them to heal tissues, regulate hormones, and boost immunity. They're safe, natural, and support your body's healing processes. |
| **Action Step:** Choose peptides under guidance from an integrative health practitioner, focusing on reputable sources and high-quality formulations to naturally enhance your health. | |

| | |
|---|---|
| Peptides are only useful for athletes or bodybuilders | Peptides benefit everyone, from those seeking relief from chronic disease and inflammation to people aiming for improved mental clarity, energy, immune function, and healthy aging. |
| **Action Step:** Identify your specific health goals (immunity, inflammation reduction, energy), and explore appropriate peptides like collagen peptides, BPC-157, or growth hormone-releasing peptides tailored to your needs. | |

| | |
|---|---|
| Peptides alone will solve chronic health issues without lifestyle changes. | Peptides are powerful tools but must be combined with a healthy lifestyle (proper nutrition, movement, sleep, and stress |

| | management) to effectively reverse chronic diseases and optimize health. |
|---|---|
| **Action Step:** Pair your peptide regimen with foundational health habits like a nutrient-rich diet, regular movement, and daily mindfulness practices for optimal results. | |

## How Do Peptides Work?

Peptides are powerful signaling molecules naturally produced by the body, acting as messengers that **enhance cellular communication and promote healing.** Here's **how** peptides support health and accelerate the body's natural recovery process:

### 1. Stimulate Growth Hormones:

- Peptides trigger the release of growth hormones, essential for tissue repair, regeneration, and cellular renewal. By activating these growth factors, peptides help accelerate healing, increase muscle mass, and improve overall recovery.

### 2. Reduce Inflammation:

- Certain peptides possess strong anti-inflammatory properties, helping the body manage inflammation more effectively. By reducing inflammation, peptides alleviate pain and create an optimal environment for healing, particularly in conditions like arthritis, chronic pain, and autoimmune diseases.

## 3. Promote Tissue Regeneration:

- Peptides such as BPC-157 and TB-500 stimulate the formation of new blood vessels, improving circulation and supplying injured tissues with essential nutrients and oxygen. This enhances tissue repair, strengthens tendons, muscles, and bones, and reduces recovery time after injuries.

## 4. Repair Injured Cells:

- Some peptides directly target specific cellular receptors, enabling injured cells to repair themselves. They rebuild structural components within tissues, facilitate regeneration of damaged cells, and enhance the body's overall capacity to recover and rebuild.

## 5. Increase Cell Migration and Repair:

- Certain peptides help cells migrate effectively to sites of injury or inflammation, accelerating the healing process. This targeted action enables quicker recovery, especially after injury, surgery, or intense physical exertion.

By harnessing the natural healing power of peptides, *you* can dramatically improve recovery, optimize health, and reclaim a life of vitality and well-being.

## Action Steps: How to Get Started with Peptides Today

Peptides offer a natural, sustainable alternative that empowers your body's innate healing mechanisms, potentially freeing you from lifelong medication dependency and costly treatments. If you want to integrate peptides into your health journey, consider these action steps today:

### STEP 1: Research & Educate Yourself
- Read credible sources like PubMed, Nature, and reputable integrative medical websites to deepen your understanding of peptides.

### STEP 2: Consult a Specialist
- Find a qualified functional medicine practitioner or integrative doctor experienced in peptide therapy.

### STEP 3: Choose Your Peptides Wisely
- Select peptides based on your health needs. Start with widely studied peptides like BPC-157, TB-500, or collagen peptides.

**STEP 4: Start Slow & Monitor**

- Begin gradually and closely monitor your body's response. Adjust dosage and type as guided by your healthcare professional.

**STEP 5: Combine with Healthy Habits**

- Pair peptide therapy with a nutrient-rich diet, consistent movement, stress management, and proper sleep to amplify benefits.

**STEP 6: Track Your Progress**

- Keep a wellness journal or log to document improvements in energy, recovery, inflammation, mood, and overall health.

Your body knows how to heal; you just need to give it the right tools. Peptides provide your body with targeted instructions to regenerate and recover, bringing you back to vibrant health. **Let peptides unlock the healing you deserve.** I have personally witnessed the incredible transformations peptides can offer. Trust your biology, trust the science, and above all, trust yourself. You've got this. Your vibrant health journey starts *now*.

## Next Up

In **Chapter 17**, we'll explore how wearable health technology and biohacking can further optimize your health and longevity

# Chapter 17:

## Biohacking Your Health: Technology for Peak Performance

Did You Know? Wearable Tech Users Reduce Chronic Disease Risk by 30%

**A study in The Lancet Digital Health found that individuals using wearable health trackers improved their metabolic health by 30%, had significantly better sleep, and were more likely to prevent chronic disease.**

Advancements in technology are revolutionizing healthcare, making it more accessible, personalized, and proactive. Wearable devices, continuous glucose monitors, and at-home lab tests now offer real-time insights into key health markers such as blood sugar levels, heart rate variability, sleep quality, and brain activity. The most significant breakthrough? You no longer have to wait for symptoms to arise. These tools empower you to identify imbalances early, optimize your health, and prevent disease before it begins.

For years, David dismissed his constant fatigue, brain fog, and high blood pressure as just part of aging. His doctor reassured him that everything was "normal for his age." But when a friend suggested he try a **Continuous Glucose Monitor (CGM),** he discovered a hidden problem: his blood sugar was spiking dangerously high after meals, even when he ate what he thought were "healthy" foods. Armed with real-time data, David made small dietary adjustments and saw immediate improvements. Within weeks, his blood sugar stabilized, his energy returned, and he lost 25 pounds, completely avoiding the diabetes diagnosis his doctor had predicted. David's story proves that **knowledge is power**. With the right tools, *you* can take control of your health before problems arise.

Your health is like flying a plane, and wearable technology is your cockpit dashboard. A pilot wouldn't fly blind without tracking altitude, speed, or fuel; just as you shouldn't navigate your health without monitoring key biomarkers. Wearable devices provide real-time insights into heart rate, sleep quality, glucose levels, and stress responses, acting as your personal flight instruments. Biohacking is your turbulence control system, allowing you to make small adjustments that optimize performance and keep you on course for longevity, energy, and peak wellness. With **the right tools**, you're not just along for the ride; you're in *full control* of your journey.

What if you could pinpoint exactly which foods spike your blood sugar?

Know if your body is burning fat efficiently? Track the quality of your sleep and find ways to improve it? Measure your real-time stress levels and learn how to lower them instantly? This *isn't* science fiction; it's the power of wearable technology and biohacking. Are *you* ready to take control of your health and unlock your peak performance?

The traditional healthcare system is largely built around managing disease after it occurs, rather than preventing it in the first place. It operates on a reactive model, treating symptoms instead of addressing the root causes before they develop.

- Waiting **until** you get sick.
- Prescribing medications to **"manage"** symptoms.
- **Ignoring** lifestyle optimization and early warning signs.

| Conventional Approach | Root-Cause Approach |
|---|---|
| Wait until symptoms appear | Track real-time biomarkers to prevent disease |
| Prescribe medications | Use biohacking tools to correct imbalances naturally |

| | |
|---|---|
| Guesswork based on outdated guidelines | Use personalized, real-time data from wearables |
| Treat chronic disease once it develops | Optimize longevity and peak performance before issues start |

Wearable health tech and biohacking allow **you** to detect and correct health problems long before they turn into chronic disease. The future of medicine is **prevention**. The question is: will you embrace it?

# Myths vs. Truths About Wearable Tech & Biohacking

| Myth | Truth |
|---|---|
| Wearable tech is just for elite athletes. | Everyday people use CGMs, sleep trackers, and HRV monitors to prevent disease and optimize health. |
| **Action Step:** Start with a wearable that tracks sleep or glucose to identify hidden health issues. ||

| | |
|---|---|
| Sleep trackers aren't accurate. | While not perfect, wearables like the Oura Ring provide valuable insights that help improve sleep quality. |

| **Action Step:** Track your sleep patterns for one week and adjust habits based on data. |
| --- |

| Biohacking is just a fad. | Cold plunges, red light therapy, and molecular hydrogen have scientific backing proving their benefits for longevity and performance. |
| --- | --- |
| **Action Step:** Experiment with one biohack (cold exposure, infrared sauna, or grounding) and track the results. | |

## How Technology is Reshaping Health

Imagine being able to predict a blood sugar spike before it happens, track your sleep cycles to optimize rest, or know exactly when your body needs hydration. This isn't the future; it's happening now. The rise of wearable health technology has created a new era of precision medicine, allowing people to make informed decisions about their health in real time.

**The latest advancements include:**

- **Continuous Glucose Monitors (CGMs)**: Track blood sugar levels and optimize diet in real time.

- **Smartwatches & Health Apps**: Monitor heart rate variability (HRV), stress, sleep, and activity levels.

- **Oura Rings**: Provide deep insights into sleep quality and recovery.

- **Biometric Patches**: Measure electrolyte balance, hydration, and metabolic function.

- **Neurofeedback Headbands**: Optimize focus, stress resilience, and cognitive performance.

# Biohacking: The Most Effective Tools for Longevity & Performance

Biohacking is the practice of using science, technology, and lifestyle changes to optimize the body's performance, health, and longevity. Biohacking empowers individuals to take control of their health by leveraging data and personalized strategies to achieve peak performance and longevity. Some examples of effective biohacking include:

**Cold Plunge Therapy:**
- Activates brown fat, boosts metabolism, and reduces inflammation.
- Improves mental resilience and mood by increasing dopamine levels.

**Red Light Therapy (Photobiomodulation):**

- Stimulates mitochondrial function for enhanced energy production.
- Accelerates tissue repair, reduces joint pain, and enhances skin health.
- Used by NASA for muscle recovery in astronauts.

**Molecular Hydrogen Therapy:**

- One of the most powerful antioxidants, reducing oxidative stress.
- Supports brain function, reduces inflammation, and improves metabolic health.
- Available in hydrogen-rich water or inhalation therapy.

**Hyperbaric Oxygen Therapy (HBOT):**

- Increases oxygen supply to tissues, accelerating healing & reducing inflammation.
- Shown to support brain function in conditions like traumatic brain injuries (TBIs) and cognitive decline.

**Infrared Sauna Therapy:**

- Promotes detoxification through sweat while reducing inflammation and improving circulation.
- Enhances cardiovascular health and longevity markers.

**Grounding (Earthing):**

- Reduces inflammation by reconnecting with the Earth's natural electrical charge.
- Shown to improve sleep, lower stress hormones, and support heart rate variability (HRV).

**Micro-circulation:**

- Enhances circulation, increases oxygen and reduces muscle spasms.
- Reduces minor pain.

# How to Integrate Wearable Tech & Biohacking into Your Life

1. **Start with Wearable Data:**
   - Use a CGM for 2 weeks to understand blood sugar trends.
   - Track HRV and sleep with an Oura Ring or smartwatch.

2. **Enhance Recovery & Performance:**
   - Try cold plunges or infrared sauna post-exercise.
   - Use red light therapy for cellular repair and skin health.

3. **Optimize Brain Function:**
   - Experiment with neurofeedback devices or molecular hydrogen.
   - Practice grounding and meditation to reduce stress.

4. **Track and Adjust:**
   - Use a biometric patch or smartwatch to measure hydration and stress.
   - Adjust diet, fasting windows, and exercise based on wearable insights.

*Any technology recommendations are intended to support general wellness and are not meant to diagnose, treat, or prevent any disease. Consult your healthcare provider before starting any new technologies.

# Your 30-Day Action Plan: Biohacking & Wearable Tech

Wearable health technology and biohacking tools are giving individuals unprecedented control over their health, optimizing performance, recovery, and longevity. Consider this step-by-step, week-by-week action plan to introduce biohacking & wearable tech into your daily life:

**WEEK 1:** Wear a CGM or Oura Ring to track baseline metrics.

**WEEK 2:** Start incorporating cold plunges or sauna therapy for cellular repair.

**WEEK 3:** Introduce red light therapy and grounding for anti-inflammatory benefits.

**WEEK 4:** Fine-tune sleep, stress management, and hydration strategies using biometric data.

**Action Step:** Choose **one** biohacking tool or wearable today and start tracking your health.

We are entering a new era, where individuals have more control over their health than ever before. Fasting, movement, nutrition, and mindset are powerful tools. **But when combined with wearable tech and biohacking,** you can accelerate healing, optimize performance, and prevent disease. I have seen that by leveraging technology and biohacking strategies, you can take full control of your health, longevity, and performance.

**Are you ready to become the CEO of your own health? The future is now.**

## Next Up

In **Chapter 18**, we'll dive deeper into Precision Health and explore how personalizing our healthcare choices, based on individual biology, genetics, lifestyle, and environment, makes our journey to lasting health more effective, efficient, and sustainable.

Chapter 18:

# Precision Health: Why Personalized Wellness Matters

Did You Know? 90% of Chronic Disease is Lifestyle-Driven, Not Genetic

**A study in the Journal of the American Medical Association found that only 10% of chronic diseases are truly genetic, meaning 90% of health outcomes are shaped by lifestyle, environment, and personal choices.**

Mainstream healthcare often relies on a one-size-fits-all approach, overlooking the fact that every individual's body is unique. Now, imagine having a personalized health plan tailored specifically to your genetics, metabolism, and lifestyle, rather than relying on generic advice. That's the transformative power of **Precision Natural Health**, a customized approach that targets your specific needs to optimize your well-being.

For years, Sarah struggled with unexplained fatigue, weight gain, and digestive issues, feeling defeated despite trying every diet, including keto, paleo, low-fat, without success. Her doctors dismissed her concerns, telling her that her lab results were normal and suggesting she simply eat fewer calories and exercise more. But when Sarah decided to take matters into her own hands with a gut microbiome test and Continuous Glucose Monitor (CGM), she uncovered the truth.

Her "healthy" morning smoothie was causing blood sugar spikes higher than soda. She also had a gut imbalance that hindered nutrient absorption, and her cortisol levels were too high, keeping her body in fat-storage mode. By making **personalized adjustments**, Sarah lost 30 pounds, healed her digestion, and regained energy, *without* starving herself.

Your health is like a custom-tailored suit, and when it's designed specifically for you, it fits perfectly, allowing you to move freely and comfortably. But when mass-produced, it's often uncomfortable, restrictive, and ineffective. Just as no two people are the same, no two bodies have identical nutritional needs, exercise responses, or metabolic functions.

Precision natural health is about creating a wellness plan that's personalized to your unique biology, rather than forcing you into a one-size-fits-all approach.

**Using genetic insights, personalized nutrition, and functional medicine**, you craft a plan that's tailored *just for you*, not the average person. By investing in a custom approach, you unlock *your* health's full potential and thrive in ways that generic solutions can never offer.

Imagine knowing exactly: Which foods fuel your body best, and which ones sabotage it. How your genetics impact weight loss, hormone balance, and longevity. The best exercise routine for **your** body. So you stop wasting time on methods that don't work. How to use wearable tech and lab tests to catch potential health issues before they start. *You* are the scientist of your own body.

**Are you ready to unlock the most optimized, energized, and healthiest version of yourself?**

Much of mainstream medicine is structured around symptom management, not health optimization. This often keeps patients cycling through treatments instead of moving toward true healing.

Doctors are often trained to treat symptoms with medication, rather than explore the deeper root causes.
Insurance models tend to support standardized care over personalized, preventive approaches.

And the broader system, including food and pharmaceutical industries, is not always aligned with long-term wellness.

This is why being informed and proactive is essential.

| Conventional Approach | Root-Cause Approach |
|---|---|
| One-size-fits-all health advice | Health plans customized to your genetics & metabolism |
| Treats symptoms after disease appears | Prevents disease before it starts |
| Uses prescription drugs to manage conditions | Uses lifestyle, nutrition, and biohacking for true healing |
| Ignores food as medicine | Uses personalized nutrition based on microbiome and metabolic health |

**The reality?** You can take charge of your health **before** disease starts. That's what Precision Natural Health is all about.

# Myths vs. Truths About Personalized Health

| Myth | Truth |
|------|-------|
| DNA determines your health; you can't change it. | Epigenetics proves that lifestyle changes can "turn off" disease-related genes. |
| **Action Step:** Start tracking how food, sleep, and stress affect your energy and mood. | |

| Myth | Truth |
|------|-------|
| All carbs and fat are the same for everyone. | Some people thrive on a high-fat ketogenic diet, while others need more carbs for energy. |
| **Action Step:** Use a CGM for 2 weeks to track which foods spike your blood sugar. | |

| Myth | Truth |
|------|-------|
| Exercise is just about burning calories. | Your body responds uniquely to different types of movement: some need more strength training; others need more cardio. |
| **Action Step:** Experiment with different workouts and track heart rate variability (HRV) to see what works best. | |

# Why One-Size-Fits-All Health Advice Doesn't Work

For decades, mainstream health advice has emphasized universal recommendations: low-fat diets, calorie restriction, and generalized workout plans. However, emerging research shows that individuals process nutrients, respond to exercise, and metabolize medications differently based on their genetic and biochemical makeup. Other variables include:

- **Different Metabolisms:** Some people thrive on a low-carb diet, while others feel fatigued and sluggish.

- **Variability in Exercise Response:** One person may build muscle quickly with strength training, while another needs more aerobic activity to improve cardiovascular health.

- **Nutrient Absorption Differences:** Some individuals absorb vitamins like B12 or D more efficiently, while others require supplementation.

A groundbreaking study published in *Cell* demonstrated that even identical meals can cause vastly different blood sugar responses in different individuals.

This highlights the need for **customized health plans** rather than generalized guidelines.

# The Role of Functional Medicine in Reversing Disease

Functional medicine focuses on identifying and addressing the root causes of health issues, rather than just masking symptoms. Unlike traditional medicine, which often relies on medications to manage disease, functional medicine aims to optimize health by looking at the whole person, considering factors like nutrition, lifestyle, genetics, and environmental influences. By targeting the underlying dysfunctions, functional medicine empowers the body's natural ability to heal, helping prevent chronic diseases and promoting long-term well-being.

**Core Principles of Functional Medicine:**

1. **Personalized Treatment**: Each patient receives an individualized plan based on genetic testing, biomarkers, and lifestyle analysis.

2. **Addressing Root Causes**: Instead of suppressing symptoms, functional medicine looks at gut health, inflammation, hormonal balance, and nutrient deficiencies to correct imbalances.

3. **Food as Medicine**: Recognizing that dietary interventions can reverse metabolic disorders, autoimmune diseases, and cardiovascular conditions.

For example, studies from *The American Journal of Clinical Nutrition* have found that dietary interventions tailored to an individual's specific gut microbiome can significantly reduce inflammation and improve metabolic health.

## How to Tailor Your Diet, Exercise, and Supplements to YOUR Body's Needs

Thanks to advancements in health technology, creating a personalized health plan is easier than ever. Here's a step-by-step guide:

1. Customizing Your Diet:

- **Monitor Blood Sugar Response**: Using a continuous glucose monitor (CGM) helps track real-time reactions to foods and optimize carbohydrate intake.

- **Assess Food Sensitivities**: Symptoms like bloating, fatigue, and brain fog can stem from undiagnosed food intolerances. Elimination diets and food sensitivity tests can provide clarity.

- **Optimize Macros Based on Metabolism**: Some people thrive on a ketogenic diet, while others do better with a balanced Mediterranean diet rich in healthy fats and lean proteins.

2. Designing an Exercise Plan for Your Body Type:

- **Genetic testing** can reveal whether you're more suited to endurance training or high-intensity workouts.
- **Heart rate variability (HRV) monitoring** helps determine recovery needs and optimal workout intensity.
- **Strength vs. Cardio Balance**: Some individuals require more strength training for bone density, while others benefit from aerobic exercise for heart health.

3. Targeted Supplementation Based on Deficiencies:

- **Vitamin D & Omega-3 Testing**: Many people are deficient in these essential nutrients, which play critical roles in immune function and inflammation control.

- **Gut Health Analysis**: Stool testing can identify imbalances in gut bacteria, guiding probiotic and prebiotic recommendations.

- **Methylation & B-Vitamins**: Genetic testing can reveal methylation issues that impact energy levels and detoxification, guiding the need for methylated B vitamins.

## Cutting-Edge Testing and Tools to Assess Your Metabolic Health

Thanks to advancements in health technology, individuals now have access to tools that provide real-time insights into their metabolic health. These innovations empower people to make informed lifestyle changes on their own. Some of these include:

### 1. Continuous Glucose Monitors (CGMs):

- CGMs provide real-time feedback on how different foods impact blood sugar, helping individuals make smarter dietary choices.

### 2. Genetic and Epigenetic Testing:

- Identifies genetic predispositions to obesity, inflammation, or cardiovascular disease.

- Reveals how lifestyle factors affect gene expression, helping individuals prevent disease before it starts.

## 3. Microbiome Testing:

- Analyzes gut bacteria composition, guiding dietary recommendations that support digestion, immune function, and mental health.

## 4. Heart Rate Variability (HRV) and Wearable Devices:

- **HRV tracking** measures stress resilience and recovery needs, guiding fitness and sleep optimization.

- **Oura Rings, Whoop Bands, and Smartwatches** provide valuable insights into sleep cycles, recovery, and metabolic rate.

*Any nutritional, supplement or technology recommendations are intended to support general wellness and are not meant to diagnose, treat, or prevent any disease. Consult your healthcare provider before starting any new supplements or technologies.

# Your 30-Day Action Plan: Precision Natural Health Challenge

While conventional health advice provides general guidelines, it often fails to account for individual differences in genetics, metabolism, and lifestyle. This is where precision health comes in, a revolutionary approach that tailors health strategies to an individual's unique biological needs. To help you take control of your health and customize your wellness routine, follow this structured plan:

### WEEK 1: Identify & Track Your Baseline

- Use a **CGM or food journal** to track how different meals affect energy.

- Monitor **HRV, sleep, and movement** with a wearable device.

- Eliminate **processed foods** and note energy changes.

### WEEK 2: Optimize Your Diet & Exercise

- Adjust your **macronutrient ratios** (low-carb, Mediterranean, keto) and track your body's response.

- Incorporate **HRV-guided exercise** for improved recovery.

- Start a **personalized supplement** routine based on deficiencies.

**WEEK 3: Fine-Tune Lifestyle & Stress Management**

- Try **breathwork, meditation, or cold exposure** for stress reduction.

- Adjust sleep habits based on **wearable tracker data.**

- Improve **gut health** through probiotic-rich foods.

**WEEK 4: Implement Long-Term Precision Health Strategies**

- Work with a **functional medicine doctor** for advanced testing.

- Establish a **long-term exercise and fasting routine.**

- Fine-tune diet based on **personalized health data.**

**Action Step:** Start tracking your health data today. Small changes lead to life-changing results!

Precision health is the future of medicine, allowing individuals to take control of their health through personalized, science-backed strategies. I have seen that by understanding your unique biology, you can optimize your diet, exercise, and lifestyle for peak performance, longevity, and well-being. **Your health is an investment, not an expense.** Don't settle for generic advice. Your body is unique. Treat it that way.

**Next Up**

In **Chapter 19**, we'll explore the role of chiropractic care in holistic healing and disease prevention.

# Chapter 19:

# Align Your Spine: Chiropractic's Role in Healing

Did You Know? 90% of Disease is Linked to Nervous System Dysfunction

**A study published in the Journal of Clinical Medicine found that spinal misalignments and nerve dysfunction contribute to chronic conditions like metabolic disorders, autoimmune diseases, and heart disease.**

Most people only think about their spine when they're in pain. But what if optimizing your spinal health could enhance digestion, sleep, immunity, and energy levels?

Mark had lived with chronic back pain and migraines for years. He tried painkillers, which only masked the problem, and countless stretching routines that brought little relief. Doctors suggested surgery as his only option. But after just a few months of chiropractic care, his migraines vanished, the pain was gone, and for the first time in years, he could exercise, sleep soundly, and think clearly. Mark realized his body **wasn't** broken; it just needed the **right adjustments** to heal itself.

Imagine living without pain, bursting with energy, and feeling completely connected to your body. What if the source of your fatigue, brain fog, or inflammation was nerve interference in your spine? What if improving your spinal health could enhance your digestion, immune function, and metabolism? What if *you* could tap into your body's natural healing abilities and take control of *your* health? This is your chance to become the hero of your own wellness journey.

Your spine is like the circuit breaker of your body: when it's wired correctly, energy flows effortlessly, but when there's interference, everything starts to malfunction. Just like a home's electrical system powers all your devices, **your spine acts as the central hub for the nerve signals that regulate every function in your body.** When the circuit breaker is overloaded or misaligned, lights flicker, devices malfunction, and systems break down. Similarly, when your spine is out of alignment, nerve signals are disrupted, leading to pain, inflammation, and dysfunction throughout your body.

Chiropractic care acts as a skilled electrician, restoring proper alignment and ensuring that the body's energy flows smoothly, allowing you to function, heal, and thrive as you were meant to.

- Doctors prescribe painkillers and anti-inflammatory drugs **instead of restoring spinal alignment.**
- Surgery is pushed as the only solution, even when **non-invasive methods exist.**
- Insurance covers medications but often **refuses to pay for holistic care.**

| Conventional Approach | Root-Cause Approach |
|---|---|
| Uses painkillers to mask symptoms | Restores spinal alignment to treat the root cause |
| Recommends surgery for back pain | Uses non-invasive adjustments to promote healing |
| Ignores nervous system health | Focuses on optimizing brain-body communication |
| Treats each symptom separately | Addresses whole-body health through spinal care |

**The truth?** You can take control of your spinal health before it gets to the point of no return.

# Myths vs. Truths About Chiropractic Care

| Myth | Truth |
|---|---|
| Chiropractic care is only for back pain. | Spinal health affects digestion, immunity, hormone balance, and energy levels. |
| **Action Step:** Evaluate your posture and notice any tension; your body may be signaling a deeper issue. ||

| Myth | Truth |
|---|---|
| Chiropractic adjustments are dangerous. | Studies show chiropractic care is safer than long-term painkillers or surgery. |
| **Action Step:** Schedule a consultation with a licensed chiropractor to assess spinal health. ||

| Myth | Truth |
|---|---|
| Once you start chiropractic care, you have to go forever. | Many people continue care because they feel better; but you decide your own treatment plan. |
| **Action Step:** Try chiropractic for one month and track your energy, sleep, and mobility. ||

# The Science of How Spinal Health Affects Chronic Disease

Your spinal health directly impacts the following:

- **Metabolism & Weight Regulation**: Nerve compression can affect the way your body burns fat and processes energy. A 2020 study in *Obesity Reviews* found that spinal misalignments can impair metabolism, leading to insulin resistance and weight gain.

- **Immune Function**: Proper nerve function strengthens the immune response, making you more resilient to fighting off infections and disease.

- **Inflammation & Pain Management**: Subluxations trigger chronic inflammation, worsening conditions like arthritis, heart disease, and autoimmune disorders. A 2021 study in *Pain Medicine* found that patients receiving chiropractic care had significantly lower levels of inflammatory markers.

- **Hormonal Balance**: Spinal misalignments can increase stress hormones (cortisol) and disrupt hormonal equilibrium.

A study published in *The Journal of Manipulative and Physiological Therapeutics* found that chiropractic adjustments help regulate nervous system function, reducing pain, inflammation, and metabolic disorders. This highlights why **maintaining spinal alignment is essential for whole-body health**.

## How to Integrate Spinal Health into Your Daily Routine

Even if you're not seeing a chiropractor yet, there are simple steps you can take today to support your spinal health and nervous system function. Paying attention to these small habits daily can make a big difference in preventing issues down the road and improving your overall well-being.

### 1. Improve Posture:

- Keep **shoulders back, head aligned, and feet flat** when sitting.
- Avoid long hours of **screen time without breaks**.
- Use **ergonomic chairs** or a standing desk.

### 2. Daily Mobility & Spinal Stretches:

- **Cat-Cow Stretch**: Improves spinal flexibility.

- **Thoracic Extension Stretch**: Reduces hunching and improves posture.
- **Hip Flexor Stretch**: Relieves lower back tension.

### 3. Hydrate & Nourish Spinal Discs:

- **Drink at least 8-10 glasses of water daily** to keep spinal discs hydrated.
- **Eat collagen-rich foods** (bone broth, fish, leafy greens) for joint health.

### 4. Reduce Stress & Support the Nervous System:

- **Practice deep breathing** to calm the nervous system.
- **Try meditation or biofeedback** to balance cortisol levels.
- **Engage in low-impact exercise** like yoga or swimming.

# Your 30-Day Action Plan: Chiropractic & Spinal Health Challenge

The nervous system plays a central role in chronic disease prevention and healing, yet it is often overlooked. Chiropractic care is one of the most powerful, non-invasive ways to optimize nervous system function, reduce inflammation, and improve metabolic health. Ready to take control of your **spinal and nervous system health**? Follow this 30-day roadmap:

**WEEK 1: Build Awareness & Daily Habits**

- Assess your posture throughout the day.

- Start a **5-minute morning spinal mobility routine.**

- Increase **water intake** to hydrate spinal discs.

**WEEK 2: Strengthen & Align the Spine**

- Add **10 minutes of spinal stretches** to your routine.

- Avoid prolonged sitting; stand up **every hour.**

- Reduce screen time before bed to support nervous system function.

**WEEK 3: Optimize Nervous System Function**

- **Schedule a chiropractic appointment.**

- Try **deep breathing or guided meditation** for stress management.
- Start core-strengthening exercises to support spinal stability.

**WEEK 4: Maintain & Track Progress**

- Reflect on how you feel after 30 days of spinal care.
- Keep up with **chiropractic adjustments or self-care habits.**
- Continue **hydration, mobility, and posture habits** for long-term benefits.

**Action Step:** Start today. Your spine is your foundation for lifelong health!

Chiropractic care isn't *just* about pain relief; it's about optimizing the nervous system for overall well-being. **The spine controls every function in the body,** and by prioritizing spinal health, you're unlocking your body's natural ability to heal, reduce inflammation, and prevent chronic disease. I have seen that by integrating chiropractic adjustments, spinal mobility, and nervous system support, you're investing in lifelong health and vitality. Take control *today*; your future self will thank you.

**Next Up:**

In **Chapter 20**, we'll talk about healthy eating, food sourcing and the power of regenerative farming on our overall health.

Chapter 20:

# Healing From the Soil Up: Why Regenerative Farming May Be the Solution

Did You Know? Over 90% of our soils are depleted of essential nutrients due to industrial farming practices.

**A landmark report from the United Nations Food and Agriculture Organization (FAO) warns that at our current rate of soil degradation, we have fewer than 60 harvests left before the world's soils can no longer support food production.**

Every bite of food we take either nourishes our bodies or further starves our cells. Just a few years ago, Jennifer, a young mother of two, faced chronic fatigue, autoimmune issues, and declining health. Doctors prescribed medication after medication, but nothing helped. Feeling desperate, she turned to nutrition, discovering **regenerative farming and food tracing.**

Within months of switching to nutrient-rich, traceable foods grown in regenerated soils, her health transformed. Jennifer went from barely surviving to thriving, *reversing* her symptoms and *reclaiming* her life.

Picture yourself at a crucial crossroads. One path leads to vitality, resilience, and long-term health through nutrient-rich, sustainably grown food. The other leads to chronic illness, fatigue, and reliance on pharmaceuticals.

The choice is yours.

By supporting regenerative farming and transparent food sourcing, you're not just improving your health; you're transforming the world.

Think of regenerative agriculture as restoring a faded masterpiece. Years of neglect and mistreatment have dulled its colors and hidden its brilliance. With careful restoration, the vibrant details reemerge. In the same way, regenerating our soils replenishes vital nutrients, unlocking our body's full potential for health and vitality.

By healing the soil, we heal ourselves. It's time to reclaim our food and restore our health!

Our current healthcare system thrives on managing chronic illness rather than curing it. The more nutrient-depleted food we eat, the more illness grows, creating lifetime pharmaceutical customers. By contrast, regenerative farming aims at the root of health, preventing disease rather than merely managing symptoms.

| Conventional Agriculture | Regenerative Agriculture |
|---|---|
| Relies on synthetic chemicals | Builds healthy soils naturally |
| Depletes nutrients from food | Restores nutrient density |
| Promotes chronic disease | Supports long-term wellness |
| Prioritizes yield over quality | Balances yield and nutrition |
| Creates dependence on pharmaceuticals | Reduces chronic health issues |

## Myths vs. Truths About Regenerative Farming

| Myth | Truth |
|---|---|
| Regenerative farming can't produce enough food. | Regenerative practices often yield comparable or greater productivity long-term by improving soil fertility and ecosystem resilience. |
| **Action Step:** Buy regenerative products to encourage market demand and scale-up production. ||

| | |
|---|---|
| Regenerative food is too expensive and unrealistic for average families. | Regenerative farming reduces reliance on expensive inputs like |

| | fertilizers and pesticides, ultimately lowering costs over time. |
|---|---|
| **Action Step:** Choose local regenerative foods, join community-supported agriculture (CSA), or farmers' markets to save money. | |

| Organic and regenerative are the same thing. | Organic can still degrade soils; regenerative goes beyond organic by actively restoring ecosystems. |
|---|---|
| **Action Step:** Look for regenerative certifications or blockchain-traced products that verify sustainability practices. | |

# How Regenerative Farming & Blockchain Revolutionize Our Food System

Regenerative farming restores soil health and boosts nutrient-rich food production, while blockchain ensures transparency and trust in the supply chain. Together, they create a more sustainable, ethical, and resilient food system that benefits both people and the planet. Here are some other reasons these processes are so important to our food and health:

- **Nutrient-Dense Foods:** Healthy soil leads directly to healthier food, richer in minerals and antioxidants vital to fighting chronic disease.

- **Operational Resilience:** Healthy soils retain water better, reducing the risks of drought and flooding, and improving the overall stability of food supply.

- **Economic Sustainability:** Farmers practicing regenerative agriculture use fewer synthetic inputs, making farming profitable and sustainable long-term.

- **Transparency & Trust:** Blockchain tracking empowers consumers to verify regenerative practices directly, ensuring transparency and authenticity.

# Your 30-Day Action Plan: Regenerative Food Challenge:

We are in charge of what we feed our bodies, and that means *we* get to decide the path that leads to good health or the one that leads to chronic disease.

Nutrition is hard to master, consider this step-by-step, week-by-week accessible action plan to help get you started today:

## WEEK 1: Educate Yourself

- Research regenerative farms in your region.
- Watch documentaries or read articles on soil regeneration.

## WEEK 2: Transition Your Shopping

- Replace one meal per day with regenerative or locally sourced foods.
- Visit a local farmers' market or join a CSA program.
- Get to know a local farmer's origin story.

## WEEK 3: Spread the Word

- Share your regenerative food journey on social media.
- Encourage friends and family to choose sustainable products.

## WEEK 4: Advocate for Change

- Support brands, like GROW, using blockchain for food tracing.

- Contact local businesses or restaurants about using regenerative products.

- Learn how a decentralized economy such as the Grow Blockchain increases TRUST in the knowledge you are consuming more nutritious food and how that can reward the farmers who raise or grow it.

By supporting regenerative agriculture and demanding transparency in the food supply, you are directly impacting your health, community, and the planet. Remember, every meal is an opportunity to nourish yourself and regenerate the world around you. You hold more power than you realize. Use it to transform not just your life, but the entire food system.

## Next Up

In **Chapter 21**, we'll explore our role in helping prevent chronic disease in our children and the next generation of adults.

Chapter 21:

# Healthy Kids for Life: Raising Disease-Proof Children

## Did You Know? Chronic Disease in Children is at an All-Time High

**In the last 30 years, childhood obesity has tripled. Type 2 diabetes, once rare in kids, is now diagnosed in children as young as 8 years old. Asthma, allergies, and autoimmune disorders are skyrocketing.**

Here's an alarming fact: Over 80% of chronic diseases can be prevented through lifestyle choices made during childhood. The foundation for lifelong health is established **in the first 18 years of life**. Knowing this, the real question then becomes: Are we setting up the next generation for health and success, or for disease?

For years, Sarah's son, Ethan, battled constant fatigue, skin rashes, and difficulty concentrating in school. Despite doctors prescribing medications for his allergies and digestive issues, *nothing* seemed to work. Frustrated, Sarah decided to try a different approach. She removed processed foods, artificial dyes, and excess sugar from his diet, opting instead for whole foods. She involved Ethan in meal prepping and made a habit of spending more time outdoors, playing and moving, while reducing screen time. Within just three months, Ethan's energy soared, his skin cleared up, and he no longer needed allergy medications. **Sarah realized that the "normal" modern diet was harming her child.** By going back to basics, she gave him the gift of health. Every child deserves this opportunity.

Raising a healthy child is like weaving a beautiful, unbreakable tapestry: each thread represents the habits, values, and nourishment you provide, creating a foundation of strength and resilience. From the moment they're born, children rely on their caregivers to weave together the fabric of their well-being.

Every meal made with love is a thread of nutrition. Every bedtime routine strengthens the weave of rest and recovery. Every moment of encouragement and emotional support fortifies their mental and emotional health. However, if the threads of nutrition, movement, and emotional balance are weak or missing, gaps appear in the tapestry, making it fragile and vulnerable to the wear and tear of life.

**As parents, caregivers, and role models, we are the master weavers of our children's health, ensuring each thread is**

**strong and vibrant.** In doing so, we create a lasting legacy of wellness that can be passed down through generations.

Your child's health is a story waiting to be written. Will it be one of vibrancy, energy, and resilience? Or will it be filled with doctor's visits, medications, and lifelong struggles? The good news is, you are the author of this story. As parents, we have the power to shape our children's habits, beliefs, and future health by guiding them toward choices that foster well-being.

The modern healthcare industry profits from managing disease, **not** preventing it. We must be the advocate our child needs in order to lead them away from becoming stuck in the cycle of "sickcare" in the future.

- Doctors often prescribe medications for childhood issues (ADHD, allergies, digestive disorders) **without addressing diet and lifestyle.**
- Fast-food industries market directly to kids, **creating sugar addictions early.**
- Pediatric chronic disease medications are **a billion-dollar industry.**

| Conventional Approach | Root-Cause Approach |
|---|---|
| Treats childhood obesity with medication | Prevents obesity by teaching healthy eating habits early |
| Prescribes antibiotics repeatedly for recurring infections | Strengthens the immune system through nutrition and gut health |
| Labels hyperactive kids as ADHD without looking at diet | Identifies sugar, food dyes, and nutrient deficiencies as possible causes |
| Recommends processed baby food & formula | Encourages whole, nutrient-dense foods from the start |

**The reality?** You don't have to wait for a diagnosis to change the trajectory of your child's health.

## Myths vs. Truths About Kids' Health

| Myth | Truth |
|---|---|
| Kids will grow out of bad eating habits. | Childhood eating patterns shape lifelong food preferences and metabolism. |
| **Action Step:** Involve kids in cooking so they develop a natural relationship with real food. | |

| A little sugar won't hurt. | Excess sugar fuels inflammation, behavioral issues, ADHD, and early insulin resistance. |
|---|---|
| **Action Step:** Swap processed snacks for whole-food alternatives like fruit, nuts, or yogurt. ||

| Sleep routines aren't that important. | Poor sleep disrupts hormones, increases obesity risk by 50%, and weakens immunity. |
|---|---|
| **Action Step:** Create a consistent, tech-free bedtime routine for better sleep quality. ||

## Breaking the Cycle: It Starts with Parents

Children don't just follow instructions; they model what they see. If we want our kids to grow up free from chronic disease, we must first look inward. Our mindset, beliefs, and behaviors shape the example we set for them. The choices we make today become the foundation for their health tomorrow. By prioritizing our own well-being, we not only improve our lives but also teach our children how to live healthy, vibrant lives of their own.

### The Parent Health Mirror

**Ask yourself:**

- **Do I prioritize** whole foods, movement, and mindfulness?

- **Am I emotionally** resilient, or do I model stress and burnout?

- **Do I rely on** processed convenience foods, or do I cook real meals?

- **Do I value** sleep, or do I sacrifice it for productivity?

**Mindset Shift:** Health isn't about fixing problems later; it's about **preventing disease from the start**.

The choices made in childhood create the **health trajectory of a lifetime**, and those choices start with your intentions as a parent.

## The Five Pillars of Childhood Chronic Disease Prevention

Research from *The Journal of the American Medical Association (JAMA)* and Harvard School of Public Health confirms that **childhood habits predict adult health outcomes**. The most evidence-based factors that prevent chronic disease include:

**Whole-food nutrition**: Processed foods are linked to higher rates of obesity, diabetes, and cognitive decline.

### Action Plan:

- Eliminate processed snacks, sodas, and artificial additives.
- Teach kids to see food as fuel for their body.
- Cook together; let kids explore healthy ingredients.

**Daily movement**: Active children have a 70% lower risk of obesity-related diseases.

### Action Plan:

- Prioritize outdoor play, sports, and active family activities.
- Limit screen time and encourage real-world exploration.
- Make movement a daily habit, not just exercise, but a way of life.

**Reduced sugar intake**: Excess sugar in kids is linked to behavioral disorders, ADHD, and insulin resistance.

### Action Plan:

- No screens an hour before bed.

- Keep bedrooms dark, cool, and free from distractions.
- Ensure 9 to 11 hours of sleep for kids and teens.

**Quality sleep**: Poor sleep increases obesity risk by 50% due to hormonal imbalances.

### Action Plan:
- Model mindfulness, teach deep breathing, gratitude, and journaling.
- Encourage emotional expression instead of suppressing feelings.
- Reduce over-scheduling: kids need downtime.

**Emotional health & stress reduction**: High-stress childhoods lead to greater risks of cardiovascular disease and mental illness.

### Action Plan:
- Make health an adventure, not a chore.
- Celebrate progress, not perfection.
- Teach kids to listen to how food, sleep, and movement make them feel.

By addressing these five pillars in childhood, we **equip our children with the tools to thrive for a lifetime.**

# Your 30-Day Action Plan: Family Health Challenge

Parents have the power to shape their children's long-term health. By making conscious choices now, we can help prevent chronic disease before it starts. The best approach is a family approach, which will engrain health-conscious behaviors in your children from an early age. Use this step-by-step, week-by-week roadmap to reinforce healthy habits today and every day:

**WEEK 1: Nutrition Reset**

- Swap **processed snacks** for whole-food alternatives.
- Eat **at least 3 colors of vegetables** daily.
- Reduce **sugar intake by half**. Replace juice/soda with water.

**WEEK 2: Move More, Sit Less**

- 60 minutes of **active play or family exercise daily**.
- Limit **screen time to 2 hours max** per day.
- Go on a **family hike, bike ride, or outdoor activity**.

**WEEK 3: Prioritize Sleep & Stress Management**

- Establish **consistent bedtime and wake-up routines**.
- Remove **electronics from bedrooms**.

- Practice **5 minutes of deep breathing or mindfulness** before bed.

**WEEK 4: Strengthening Family Connection**

- Eat at **least one meal together** every day with **no screens**.
- Plan **one technology-free day** as a family.
- Encourage **open conversations about health & emotions**.

**Action Step:** Cook one healthy meal together as a family this week using whole, healthy foods.

I have seen that by investing in your child's health now, you can **prevent chronic disease before it starts**. This is not about perfection: it's about progress, intention, and creating a home where wellness is a way of life. Health is not something you "fix" later. It's something you build from the start. Every meal, every bedtime routine, every outdoor adventure. It's all shaping their future. Your child's health is in *your* control. The question is: What will *you* do with that power?

## Next Up

In **Chapter 22**, we'll explore the power of social connections and how strong relationships influence long-term health.

# Chapter 22:

## The Ripple Effect: Inspiring a Healthier Community

Did you Know? Your Social Circle May be the Single Biggest Predictor of Your Health

**A study published in The New England Journal of Medicine found that if a close friend becomes obese, your chances of becoming obese increase by 57%. Even if they live far away. But here's the good news: Just as unhealthy habits spread, so do healthy ones.**

When one person in a social group adopts healthier habits: eating better, exercising, and managing stress, it naturally influences those around them, often without saying a word. Your personal transformation doesn't just improve *your* life; it sparks a ripple effect, inspiring others to make positive changes in their own lives.

By leading by example in self-health, **you can create a culture of wellness that extends far beyond yourself**, empowering everyone in your circle to thrive.

For years, Mike struggled with poor health. Overweight, exhausted, and relying on multiple medications, he felt like he had tried every diet and workout plan. But nothing worked. Worse, his family wasn't supportive. His wife brought home fast food, his kids spent hours on screens, and his friends mocked his attempts to live healthier.

One day, after yet another failed attempt at weight loss, Mike decided to stop trying to convince others. Instead, he focused on his own health. He eliminated processed foods and sugar from his diet, which his wife noticed, and started cooking healthier meals in response. He began walking daily, and soon his kids asked to join him for bike rides. He cut back on weekend drinking, and his friends respected his decision, some even joining in.

Within six months, Mike lost 50 pounds, his energy soared, and without ever pressuring anyone, his entire household began to transform. Mike's story shows that the best way to inspire change isn't by telling others what to do. It's by showing them what's possible.

Think of your health as a stone thrown into a still lake. The first ripple begins with your personal choices: what you eat, how you move, and how you manage stress.

The second ripple extends to your family: they notice your increased energy, healthier habits, and positive mindset.

The third ripple reaches your friends, coworkers, and community, as they see the transformation in you and feel inspired to make changes themselves. The more consistent your choices, the greater your impact. Your health isn't just about you; it's a legacy that can positively affect everyone around you.

By now you know that the healthcare industry is structured to manage disease rather than preventing it.

But what if we took back control? What if we stopped waiting for the system to fix us and instead build healthier communities from the ground up? That's where **you** come in.

| Conventional Approach | YOUR Approach |
|---|---|
| Encourages weight loss through medications | Encourages weight loss through real food and movement |
| Treats stress-related illnesses with anti-anxiety meds | Teaches mindfulness, sleep, and nervous system regulation |
| Focuses on treating disease after it happens | Focuses on preventing disease before it starts |
| Views health as an individual responsibility | Recognizes that health is influenced by community, environment, and habits |

**The reality?** You're in control of your health, and you have the tools to show others that they can be too.

## Myths vs. Truths About Inspiring Others to Get Healthy

| Myth | Truth |
|---|---|
| People don't change unless you push them. | People change when they are inspired, not pressured. |
| **Action Step:** Lead by example. Instead of nagging, let your energy, transformation, and vitality speak for itself. | |

| Myth | Truth |
|---|---|
| I need to wait until I'm perfect before helping others. | Progress is more inspiring than perfection. |
| **Action Step:** Share your journey, not just your success, but your struggles, too. Real people relate to real challenges. | |

| Myth | Truth |
|---|---|
| One person can't make a difference. | Every great movement in history started with ONE person. |
| **Action Step:** Decide to be the spark that ignites change in your family, workplace, and community. | |

# The Ripple Effect: How Your Health Transformation Impacts Others

I want you to think about throwing the stone into the still lake again. The ripples it creates expand **outward**, touching everything in their path. **This is what happens when you take charge of your health.** Your improved energy, vitality, and mindset influence those around you, often without you realizing it. Other ways your health journey can be impactful include:

## Leading by Example

Studies show that **health behaviors are highly contagious**. If someone in your circle starts eating healthy, exercising, and managing stress, you are more likely to do the same. When you choose healthy foods, your children, spouse, or coworkers take notice. When you prioritize movement, friends are more likely to join you for a walk or gym session. When you manage stress effectively, it creates a calmer environment for those around you.

A study published in the *International Journal of Behavioral Nutrition and Physical Activity* highlights how significantly social norms influence our health choices. It shows that when people notice their friends, family, or coworkers regularly practicing healthy habits, they perceive these behaviors as common and desirable, making them more likely to adopt similar habits themselves. This emphasizes that actions like healthy eating, regular exercise, and effective stress management can spread positively through social networks, reinforcing the contagious nature of health behaviors. Become the leader of your network of friends and co-workers.

## Encouraging Loved Ones Without Pushing

Not everyone is ready for change, but **small acts of encouragement make a difference**. Instead of preaching about diet and exercise, lead through action:

- Invite loved ones to cook a healthy meal together.
- Suggest group activities like yoga, hiking, or dance classes.
- Share books, documentaries, or podcasts that inspire without judgment.

When people see the benefits of your lifestyle (better sleep, more energy, reduced stress) on their own, without being pushed or forced to do so, they will **naturally want to follow your lead**.

# The Power of Support Groups, Accountability, and Community-Based Health Initiatives

Humans are social creatures, and our health is deeply influenced by the people we surround ourselves with. Research shows that social support is one of the strongest predictors of long-term health and behavior change.

## The Role of Accountability Partners

Having someone to check in with dramatically increases the chances of success in any health goal. A study in *The American Journal of Health Promotion* found that people who had an **accountability partner were 65% more likely to reach their health goals** compared to those who tried alone. There are several ways to establish this relationship while on your health journey, including:

- Find a workout buddy or nutrition accountability partner.
- Join an online health challenge or support group.
- Set weekly check-ins with a friend to discuss progress and struggles.

## Community-Based Health Programs

Health initiatives at the community level make wellness **accessible and engaging.** Some successful models include:

- **Farmers' markets and local food co-ops** that provide access to whole, organic foods.

- **Workplace wellness programs** offering group fitness, mental health resources, and nutrition education.

- **Church and community fitness groups**, such as walking clubs or group meditation sessions.

A 2018 study in Preventive Medicine Reports found that community-based wellness programs lead to higher participation and sustained health improvements compared to individual efforts.

# Why Reversing Chronic Disease Must Be a Collective Effort

Chronic disease is not just an individual problem; **it is a societal issue**. The rates of obesity, diabetes, heart disease, and metabolic disorders continue to rise, not because people lack willpower, but because our environment *promotes* unhealthy choices. We need to act as a community when battling chronic disease, or else we all continue to struggle.

## Shifting the Health Paradigm

We must as a society transition from a **reactive model** (treating disease after it develops) to a **preventive model** focused on:

- **Education:** Teaching people about real food, movement, and stress management.
- **Policy Change:** Advocating for better food standards, reduced sugar in processed foods, and more green spaces for activity.
- **Healthcare Reform:** Moving away from symptom management toward root-cause approaches.

## Creating a Culture of Self-Health

Self-health should be woven into the fabric of daily life, occupying as many spaces as possible for total and complete impact. These spaces include:

- **Schools:** We should be teaching nutrition, movement, and mindfulness alongside academics.

- **Workplaces:** Employee health should be prioritized through breaks, standing desks, and wellness initiatives.

- **Cities/Towns:** Investing in walkable infrastructure, parks, and fitness-friendly public spaces promote societal wellness.

A global meta-analysis in *The Lancet* concluded that if physical inactivity were reduced by just 10%, millions of lives could be saved annually. This underscores the urgency of making wellness a **collective priority**.

## Practical Action Steps to Implement Daily

**Be the Example**: Focus on your own health transformation first and let others be naturally inspired by your actions.

**Start Small with Your Family**: Swap out processed snacks, cook together, or start a daily walk as a family ritual.

**Find or Create a Support Group**: Join a fitness class, an online health community, or a local wellness meetup.

**Use Social Media for Good**: Share health tips, recipes, and success stories to encourage friends and followers.

**Advocate for Health in Your Workplace**: Suggest wellness challenges, walking meetings, or healthy office snacks.

**Get Involved in Community Health Initiatives**: Support farmers' markets, local gyms, and educational programs.

**Encourage Movement and Play**: Make fitness fun by joining a sports league, taking dance lessons, or organizing outdoor activities.

# Your 30-Day Action Plan: Community Health Challenge

**Health is contagious.** Just as disease spreads through unhealthy habits, wellness spreads through inspiration, knowledge, and collective effort. When one person transforms their health, the benefits ripple out to their family, friends, and community. Over the next month, focus on **creating a ripple effect** in your family, workplace, and community:

## WEEK 1: Inspire Your Inner Circle

- Share your **personal health journey** with close friends & family.

- Invite a **friend or family member to join a workout, yoga, or walk.**

- Swap **one unhealthy family meal for a whole-food homemade meal**.

## WEEK 2: Expand Your Reach

- Join a health-related community event, **like a farmers' market or group fitness class**.

- Start a small **family or workplace health challenge** (e.g., drink more water, move daily).

- Share a **wellness resource** (podcast, book, or documentary) with friends.

## WEEK 3: Advocate for Change

- Suggest a **workplace wellness initiative** (e.g., standing desks, walking meetings).

- Organize a **group hike, potluck with healthy foods, or meditation session**.

- Reduce **screen time** as a family and replace it with **active, social activities**.

## WEEK 4: Strengthen Community Bonds

- Introduce **a new healthy habit** to someone in your life.

- Support **local health-focused businesses** (farmers' markets, wellness centers, fitness studios).

- Reflect on **how your personal health transformation has influenced others**.

Reducing chronic disease starts with individual action, **but** its success depends on collective effort. The world doesn't change because of big institutions; it changes because of people like *you* who take action. When you take control of your health, you're not just improving your own life; you're creating a ripple effect that is felt for generations. Are you ready to be the spark?

**Next Up**

In the **final chapter**, we'll explore how to take everything learned in this book and create a personalized, sustainable plan for lifelong health and vitality. You have the power to create change, starting today.

# Conclusion:

## Taking Back Your Health, Starting Now

## Now You Know: Self-Health is Your Choice

Imagine standing at a crossroads. One path leads to chronic disease, fatigue, and a lifetime of medications. The other leads to vitality, strength, and a life free from preventable illness. The choice is *yours.*

Every decision (what you eat, how you move, how you manage stress, and how you connect with others) shapes your health journey. For too long, we've been led to believe that disease is inevitable, that aging equals decline, and that medication is the only solution. But the truth is, **most chronic illnesses are preventable**, and even reversible, through lifestyle changes.

The power to heal, thrive, and reclaim your health has always been within *you.* We live in a world where chronic disease is the norm, but it doesn't have to be your reality. The latest research has made one thing abundantly clear:
Your lifestyle has a greater impact on your long-term health than your genetics ever will:

A study in *The Lancet* found that 80% of heart disease, stroke, and Type 2 diabetes cases could be prevented through **lifestyle interventions.**

Research in *Nature Medicine* revealed that biological aging can be slowed, or even reversed, by **optimizing sleep, reducing inflammation, and maintaining metabolic health.**

A Harvard Medical School review confirmed that social connections, purpose, and mindset **play a critical role in longevity and well-being.**

The most powerful message of this book is simple:

*You are in control. Every decision you make today about your health moves you toward either a healthier tomorrow or a sicker one. Your body is designed to heal, and you already have the tools to make it happen. Make a good decision!*

## The Journey to a Disease-Free Life Starts Today

Healing doesn't happen overnight, but it starts with small, consistent steps.

Just as a single drop of water creates ripples across a pond, your daily choices accumulate into profound changes over time. Your diet fuels your future. Every bite you take is either feeding disease or fighting it.

Your movement determines your longevity. Every step you take strengthens your metabolism and prevents deterioration. Your stress levels shape your health. Every deep breath and act of mindfulness reduces inflammation and supports healing. Your mindset directs your path. Every positive thought and habit build resilience and vitality. Health is not about perfection; it's about progress.

## Self-Health Actions You Can Take NOW

If you take only one thing from this book, let it be this: You have the power to change your health, starting **today**. Here's how to begin:

### Make One Small Change Today
- Swap **one processed meal** for a whole-food alternative.
- Walk for **10 minutes after a meal** to stabilize blood sugar.

- Turn off **screens an hour before bed** to improve sleep quality.

**Set a Personal Health Goal**
- **Want to reduce inflammation?** Prioritize an anti-inflammatory diet.
- **Want to improve metabolism?** Incorporate strength training and intermittent fasting.
- **Want to increase energy?** Optimize hydration, sleep, and stress management.

**Find Accountability and Community**
- Join a **health group**, whether in person or online.
- Partner with a **friend or family member** for support and motivation.
- Share your **health journey** with others; it may inspire them to take action, too.

**Track Your Progress**
- Use a **journal or an app** to monitor your habits and improvements.
- Celebrate **milestones, no matter how small**.
- Adjust your approach based on **what works best for your body and lifestyle**.

**Commit to Lifelong Learning and Growth**

- Stay **curious**: read books, listen to podcasts, and follow evidence-based health experts.
- Experiment and **personalize your approach**; what works for one person may not work for another.
- Keep **evolving**; your health needs will change, and that's okay.

## The Final Takeaway: You Are in Control

My hope is that this book has provided you with the science, strategies, and tools you need to help you reclaim your health. **But knowledge is only powerful when put into action.** You don't have to wait for a perfect moment: start now. Every step toward health is a step toward freedom: freedom from unnecessary suffering, from preventable disease, and from limitations that hold you back from living fully.

Chronic disease is like a computer running on a corrupt operating system, glitching, running slow, and crashing. You wouldn't just keep restarting the system and expecting a different result. You need to remove the viruses (toxins, stress, poor nutrition) and reinstall a clean operating system (healthy habits, detoxification, cellular repair). Once restored, the system runs smoothly again.

If you've ever felt frustrated with your health, overwhelmed by conflicting advice, or trapped in a cycle of medications and fatigue, this book is for you. Living with a self-health attitude is your choice. Take back your health, **one day at a time.**

# Bibliography

**Chronic Disease & Epidemiology**

1. Centers for Disease Control and Prevention. (2023). *Chronic Diseases in America: The Leading Causes of Death and Disability in the United States.*

2. World Health Organization. (2022). *Noncommunicable diseases: Key facts.*

3. GBD 2019 Risk Factors Collaborators. (2020). Global burden of 87 risk factors in 204 countries, 1990–2019. *The Lancet,* 396(10258), 1223-1249.

**Nutrition & Disease Prevention**

4. Willett, W. C., & Ludwig, D. S. (2020). Dietary quality over quantity in obesity prevention and treatment. *JAMA,* 324(9), 859-860.

5. Mozaffarian, D., Rosenberg, I., & Uauy, R. (2018). Guidelines for preventing chronic disease through nutrition. *BMJ,* 361, k2396.

6. Ludwig, D. S., Hu, F. B., et al. (2018). Role of dietary carbohydrates in chronic disease. *BMJ,* 361, k2340.

**Metabolic Health & Insulin Resistance**

7. Taylor, R. (2019). Type 2 diabetes: Etiology and reversibility. *Diabetes Care*, 42(6), 1017-1025.

8. Samuel, V. T., & Shulman, G. I. (2016). Pathogenesis of insulin resistance. *Journal of Clinical Investigation*, 126(1), 12-22.

9. Hall, K. D., et al. (2019). Ultra-processed diets cause weight gain. *Cell Metabolism*, 30(1), 67-77.

**Exercise & Chronic Disease Prevention**

10. Ekelund, U., et al. (2019). Physical activity, sedentary time, and mortality. *BMJ*, 366, l4570.

11. Warburton, D. E. R., & Bredin, S. S. D. (2017). Health benefits of physical activity. *Current Opinion in Cardiology*, 32(5), 541-556.

12. Booth, F. W., et al. (2012). Exercise and chronic disease. *Comprehensive Physiology*, 2(2), 1143-1211.

**Sleep, Stress & Mental Health**

13. Walker, M. P. (2017). *Why We Sleep*. Scribner.

14. Buysse, D. J. (2014). Defining sleep health. *Sleep*, 37(1), 9-17.

15. McEwen, B. S., & Gianaros, P. J. (2011). Stress-induced brain plasticity. *Annual Review of Medicine*, 62, 431-445.

## Toxins & Environmental Health

16. Trasande, L. (2019). *Sicker, Fatter, Poorer*. Houghton Mifflin Harcourt.

17. Lanphear, B. P. (2015). Toxins and developing brain. *Annual Review of Public Health*, 36, 211-230.

18. Grandjean, P., & Landrigan, P. J. (2006). Neurotoxicity of industrial chemicals. *The Lancet*, 368(9553), 2167-2178.

## Childhood Health & Chronic Disease Prevention

19. Lustig, R. H. (2021). *Metabolical*. HarperWave.

20. Hannon, T. S., et al. (2005). Childhood obesity and diabetes. *Pediatrics*, 116(2), 473-480.

21. Skinner, A. C., et al. (2018). Prevalence of obesity in US children. *Pediatrics*, 141(3), e20173459.

## Mindset, Behavior Change & Sustainable Health Transformation

22. Prochaska, J. O., & DiClemente, C. C. (1983). Stages of change model. *Journal of Consulting and Clinical Psychology*, 51(3), 390-395.

23. Dweck, C. S. (2006). *Mindset: The New Psychology of Success*. Random House.

24. Kahneman, D. (2011). *Thinking, Fast and Slow*. Farrar, Straus and Giroux.

## Alcohol & Chronic Disease

25. National Institute on Alcohol Abuse and Alcoholism. (2023). Alcohol Facts and Statistics.

26. Centers for Disease Control and Prevention. (2022). Excessive Alcohol Use and Risks to Men's and Women's Health.

## Fasting, Autophagy, & Longevity

27. Longo, V. D., & Panda, S. (2016). Fasting, circadian rhythms, and longevity. *Cell Metabolism*, 23(6), 1048-1059.

28. Mattson, M. P., et al. (2018). Intermittent metabolic switching and neuroplasticity. *Nature Reviews Neuroscience*, 19(2), 63-80.

## Peptides & Regenerative Medicine

29. Reid, R., & Abate, J. (2022). Peptides in regenerative medicine. *Regenerative Medicine*, 17(4), 231-242.

30. Cotrim, C., & Moro, A. M. (2023). Growth hormone-releasing peptides and muscle recovery. *Journal of Clinical Endocrinology & Metabolism*, 108(1), 37-48.

## Precision Health & Personalized Medicine

31. Topol, E. (2019). *Deep Medicine: How AI Can Make Healthcare Human Again*. Basic Books.

32. Hood, L., & Friend, S. H. (2011). Predictive, personalized, preventive medicine. *Science*, 331(6015), 565-566.

**Regenerative Farming & Food Systems**

33. Montgomery, D. R., & Biklé, A. (2022). *What Your Food Ate: How to Heal Our Land and Reclaim Our Health*. W. W. Norton & Company.

34. Rodale Institute. (2020). The Power of the Plate: The Case for Regenerative Organic Agriculture in Improving Human Health.

**Wearable Health Technology & Biohacking**

35. Topol, E. (2015). *The Patient Will See You Now: The Future of Medicine Is in Your Hands*. Basic Books.

36. National Institutes of Health. (2021). Wearable Technology and Health.

**Chiropractic & Integrative Medicine**

37. Hawk, C., Schneider, M. J., et al. (2017). Best practices for chiropractic care. *Journal of Alternative and Complementary Medicine*, 23(10), 764-771.

**Mental Health & Chronic Disease**

38. National Institute of Mental Health. (2023). Mental Health and Chronic Diseases.

39. American Psychological Association. (2022). Stress in America Survey.

## Additional Sources for General Use

40. Harvard Health Publishing. (2023). Harvard Medical School: Health Guides.

41. Mayo Clinic. (2023). Comprehensive Medical Guides.

# Acknowledgements

Creating this book has truly been a journey, one supported by remarkable individuals whose contributions have been invaluable.

To my family: Karen, the love of my life, whose unwavering support and love are my constant source of strength; my incredible sons, Gianni and Luciano, who inspire me every day; my wonderful mother, Gladys, whose wisdom and guidance shaped my foundation; and my brothers, Pierluigi, Aldo, and Paolo, who have always stood by my side. Each of you has significantly contributed to my ability to bring this book to life.

To Rick Anson for your support and passion to help so many regain their health.

My heartfelt appreciation to my talented team, Rona Angeles, Cy Deangkinay, Bethel Aquino, Daria Pechaico, Michelle Abraham, Troy Lacher, and Rebecca White, your dedication, creativity, and expertise have made this project not only possible but exceptional.

To Michael Gorton, thank you for your inspiration, experience, and wisdom.

To Dr. Adam Boender, for your research and insights on Peptides.

Special thanks to T.R. McManus for providing valuable insights and research on stem cells.

To Makenzie Ozycz for your amazing editing and continued effort to push me to make this book better.

Special thanks to Shefa Rumby for the stunning cover design and impeccable formatting that brought my vision vividly to life.

Finally, to my devoted followers and colleagues who continually encourage me to share content aimed at improving humanity's health, your enthusiasm and commitment fuel my passion and purpose.

# About The Author

**Dr. Fab Mancini,** DC, FICC, FACC is a popular health and lifestyle media expert and a global voice for self-healing and preventative health. He is the international best-selling author of *The Power of Self-Healing* with Hay House and the host of the new podcast *Ending Chronic Disease*, created for those ready to take back control of their health.

He is also the host of the TV series *Thriving in the New Normal*, the popular radio show *Self-Healing with Dr. Fab*, and the podcast *The Fab Life*. Dr. Fab is a best-selling author of *Chicken Soup for the Chiropractic Soul* and has inspired millions as a world-renowned chiropractor, international speaker, educator, business leader, and President Emeritus of Parker University.

A trusted mentor to CEOs and organizations around the world, Dr. Mancini has been featured on *Dr. Phil, The Doctors,* Fox News, CNN, CBS, ABC, NBC, Univision, Telemundo, and more. He's been featured in numerous health documentaries and honored with awards including Humanitarian of the Year, CEO of the Year, Heroes for Humanity, and induction into the Wellness Revolutionaries Hall of Fame.

Dr. Mancini is a graduate of Harvard University's prestigious Institute for Educational Management and has left a global legacy in education, the Library at UNEVE, one of Mexico's top universities, proudly bears his name.

For more information and resources, visit:

http://endingchronicdisease.com or https://drfabmancini.com

www.ingramcontent.com/pod-product-compliance
Lightning Source LLC
Chambersburg PA
CBHW052120270326
41930CB00012B/2699